Handbook of

Handbook of Dermoscopy

Josep Malvehy, MD
Department of Dermatology, IDIBAPS, Barcelona, Spain

Susana Puig, MD
Department of Dermatology, IDIBAPS, Barcelona, Spain

Ralph P Braun, MD
*Department of Dermatology, University Hospital Geneva,
Geneva, Switzerland*

Ashfaq A Marghoob, MD
*Department of Dermatology, Memorial Sloan Kettering
Cancer Center, New York, USA*

Alfred W Kopf, MD, MS(Derm)
Skin and Cancer Unit, NYU Medical Center, New York, USA

informa
healthcare

New York   London

First published in 2006 by Taylor & Francis, an imprint of the Taylor & Francis Group.

This edition published in 2011 by Informa Healthcare, Telephone House, 69-77 Paul Street, London EC2A 4LQ, UK.

Simultaneously published in the USA by Informa Healthcare, 52 Vanderbilt Avenue, 7th Floor, New York, NY 10017, USA.

Informa Healthcare is a trading division of Informa UK Ltd. Registered Office: 37–41 Mortimer Street, London W1T 3JH, UK. Registered in England and Wales number 1072954.

A CIP record for this book is available from the British Library.

Library of Congress Cataloging-in-Publication Data available on application

ISBN-13: 978-0-415-38490-2

Orders may be sent to: Informa Healthcare, Sheepen Place, Colchester, Essex CO3 3LP, UK
Telephone: +44 (0)20 7017 5540
Email: CSDhealthcarebooks@informa.com
Website: http://informahealthcarebooks.com/

For corporate sales please contact: CorporateBooksIHC@informa.com
For foreign rights please contact: RightsIHC@informa.com
For reprint permissions please contact: PermissionsIHC@informa.com

Contents

Acknowledgment

Some of the images in this handbook are from the collection of the Consortium on Dermoscopic Images provided by Ralph P Braun, Armand B Cognetta, Seth Felder, Alfred W Kopf, Josep Malvehy, Ashfaq A Marghoob, Scott W Menzies, Margaret C Oliviero, Susana Puig, Harold S Rabinovitz and Steven Q Wang. The authors of this handbook are grateful for their permission to use these images.

Introduction

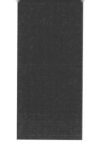

When cutaneous lesions are examined by the naked eye, many of the succinct features are obscured by reflection, refraction and diffraction of light, principally by the stratum corneum. By adding a "clearing" medium (e.g. fluid such as oil, gel or alcohol), the stratum corneum is rendered relatively transparent allowing for the visualization of structures that cannot be seen by the naked eye. The ability to visualize these structures significantly improves the in-vivo diagnostic accuracy and allows the clinician to better judge which lesions require biopsy and which do not.

The *Handbook of Dermoscopy* is designed by the editors with two principal goals in mind:

■ to provide a succinct summary coupled with a richly illustrated, comprehensive, dermoscopic atlas

■ to slip into the reader's pocket for instant availability and ease of portability.

The handbook provides high-quality images of the quintessential features and basic structures which can be identified by dermoscopy and which can be used to differentiate pigmented lesions of the skin. Thus, this microscopic technique is most helpful in assisting the clinician in the diagnosis of melanocytic neoplasms.

A rich literature has rapidly accumulated to indicate that adding dermoscopy to the clinical examination substantially improves diagnostic accuracy, which, in turn, reduces the number of biopsies, thus lowering the cost of medical care and unwanted surgical morbidity. In addition, this procedure will build not only your clinical confidence but also that of your patients.

Enjoy!!!

The authors

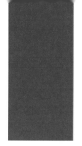

Authors' note

NB: This handbook is based on images, structures and features as seen with light emitting diode (LED) light contact dermoscopy, utilizing a liquid interface, or a dermoscope equipped with cross-polarization lens. Polarization eliminates the need for a liquid interface or direct contact with the skin. Although, most of the structures and colors seen with LED dermoscopy and polarized dermoscopy are equivalent, there are some notable differences. For those using polarized dermoscopy, it is important to note that the following structures are more difficult to appreciate under polarized light: blue-white veil; regression structures (blue-gray areas/granules, peppering); and milia-like cysts. However, milky-red areas and vascular structures are much easier to see with polarized dermoscopy. Images provided with cross-polarization lens are distinguished in the Handbook with CPL.

Structures and colors

Dermoscopic structures

- Pigment network (reticulation) (Figure A1): web-like structure consisting of brown or black lines and hypopigmented holes which create a honeycomb-like pattern. Rarely, the lines are white (reverse network).
    - Typical network: uniform, regular lines and holes, even color, fades at the periphery.
    - Atypical network: non-uniform, darker and/or broadened lines; heterogeneous holes in areas or shapes; abruptly ends at the perimeter.

- Pseudonetwork (Figures A11, A12): because the face has absent or poorly developed rete ridges, diffuse pigmentation interrupted by the surface openings of the adnexal structures (sebaceous glands, hair follicles, etc.) creates a network-like pattern.

- Structureless (Figures A3, A6) (homogeneous) areas: regions devoid of structures and without signs of regression. These areas can be pigmented or hypopigmented. However, if the area is black in color it is called a "blotch".

- Dots (Figures A5, A14): dark brown to black, brown or blue-gray, small spherical structures less than 0.1 mm diameter.

- Peppering (Figures A5, A6): tiny, blue-gray granules of melanin.

- Globules (Figures A2, A3, A5, A8, A9): brown, black or red spherical or ovoid structures with diameters usually greater than 0.1 mm.

- Cobblestone globules (Figure A2): polygonal globules crowded together causing their deformation, resulting in a cobblestone pattern.

- Radial streaming (Figure A7): linear extensions at the edge of the lesion.

- Pseudopods (Figure A3): brown-black, finger-like projections from the perimeter of the lesion. Variously-shaped knobs are present at the termini of the projections.

■ Streaks (Figures A3, A6, A7): alternate term for radial streaming and/or pseudopods. When symmetrically arranged around the entire edge of the lesion, the appellation "starburst pattern" is used.

■ Branched streaks (Figure A1): network fragments resulting from a broken-up network.

■ Blotches (Figures A3, A5–7, A9): dark brown to black, usually homogeneous, areas of pigment obscuring underlying structures. A blotch usually does not encompass the entire lesion. NB: all blotches are structureless but not all structureless areas are blotches.

■ Regression areas (Figures A5–9): white, scar-like depigmentation often combined with blue-gray peripheral zone and/or peppering (speckled blue-gray granules).

■ Blue-white veil (Figures A5, A8): irregularly marginated, confluent blue pigmentation with overlying, white, ground-glass haze.

■ Vascular structures (Figures A10, A22, A24, A27): the primary structure of hemangiomas and vascular malformations are clusters of blood vessels called "lacunae" or "saccules". Various telangiectasias of multiple shapes and sizes, including comma, pinpoint, arborizing, wreath-like, hairpin-like, irregular and glomerular.

■ Milia-like cysts (Figure A22): small, white or yellow cystic structures resembling milia which often shine brightly ("stars in the sky") when viewed with the dermoscope. Pigmented milia-like cysts can resemble brown globules.

■ Comedo-like openings (Figure A22): blackhead-like plugs due to keratin-filled invaginations on the skin surface.

■ Fingerprint-like structures (Figure A11): thin light brown parallel running lines resulting in patterns that resemble fingerprints.

■ Ridges and fissures (Figure A22): cerebriform surface resulting in gyri (ridges) and sulci (fissures). The latter can be filled with keratin-producing irregular linear, pigmented, bands.

■ "Fat fingers": broadened, hyper- or hypopigmented, digitate structures that are gyri and that can be straight, kinked, circular or branched and are seen primarily in seborrheic keratoses.

- Moth-eaten border (Figure A11): concave invaginations of the lesion border resembling defects shaped like those of the edges of a moth-eaten garment.

- Leaf-like areas (Figure A28): brown to blue-gray, discrete, structures resembling leaf-like patterns.

- Spokewheel-like structures (Figure A29): brown to gray-blue radial projections meeting at a darker brown or black central "hub".

- Large blue-gray ovoid nests (Figure A28): circumscribed, blue-gray or brown, ovoid structures larger than globules.

- Multiple blue-gray globules (Figure A27, A28): spherical, well-circumscribed structures which, in the absence of a pigment network, suggest basal-cell carcinoma.

- Parallel patterns (Figure A14, A15, A17, A18): on acral areas, parallel rows of pigmentation following the ridges or the furrows of the dermoglyphics.

- Milky-red areas (Figure A10): red-pink whitish veil resulting from increased vascularity.

- Pink-white shiny areas: seen in basal cell carcinomas.

Dermoscopic colors

Eumelanin pigment has a brown color. However, on dermoscopy, eumelanin is seen as an array of colors depending primarily on its position in the skin. Thus, eumelanin in the stratum corneum is black; in the remainder of the epidermis and upper cutis, brown; in the papillary dermis, gray; and in the lower papillary and reticular dermis, blue. When melanin is present in large quantity in several layers, the color is black.

In addition, other colors are seen on dermoscopy including: red (due to vascularity and/or inflammation); white (due to depigmentation and/or scarring); yellow (due to sebaceous material and/or hyperkeratosis); orange (due to serum resulting from erosion or superficial ulceration); jet black (due to congealed blood).

The various colors aforementioned are shown in Figure 1.1. A histopathologic correlation of the principal dermoscopic structures is shown in Table 1.1 and a schematic correlation is represented in Figure 1.2.

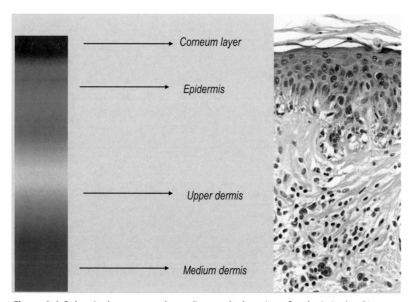

Figure 1.1 Colors in dermoscopy depending on the location of melanin in the skin.

Table 1.1 Histopathologic correlation of the principal dermoscopic structures.

Dermoscopic feature	Histopathologic correlation
Pigmentation and color	Melanin, keratin and hemoglobin at different levels in skin anatomy
Pigment network	Melanocytic pigmentation or melanin in keratinocytes along the rete ridges
Pigment pseudonetwork	Pigment in the epidermis or dermis interrupted by follicular and adnexal openings of the face
Black dots	Aggregates of melanocytes or melanin granules in the upper epidermis or stratum corneum
Multiple blue-gray dots 'peppering'	Melanophages/ melanin in the upper dermis
Brown globules	Nests of melanocytes in the upper dermis
Radial streaming and pseudopods (streaks)	Aggregates of tumor cells running parallel to the epidermis (Spitz/Reed nevi or radial growth phase of melanoma)

Table 1.1 Continued

Blue-whitish veil	Compact aggregation of heavily pigmented tumor cells in the superficial dermis in combination with compact orthokeratosis, acanthosis and more or less pronounced hypergranulosis
Blotches	Aggregates of melanin in the stratum corneum, epidermis and upper dermis
Parallel furrow pattern	Melanocytic pigmentation in the furrows on glabrous skin
Parallel ridge pattern	Melanocytic pigmentation in ridges on glabrous skin
Blue-red lagoons	Dilated vascular spaces located in the upper or mid-dermis
Vessels/erythema	Tumoral angiogenesis
Spoke-wheel areas	Nests and proliferation of pigmented basal cell carcinoma cells
Leaf-like areas	Nodules of pigmented basal cell carcinoma cells located in the upper dermis
Large ovoid blue nests	Nests of basal cell tumor in the dermis
Multiple blue globules	Nests of basal cell tumor in the dermis
White central patch	Fibrohystiocytic tumor in the dermis that is in close approximation to the epidermis
Fissures (sulci)/crypts and ridges (gyri)	Clefts and ridges seen in papillomatous tumors
Milia-like cysts	Intraepidermal keratin cysts
Follicular plugs or comedo-like openings	Comedo-like openings containing keratin

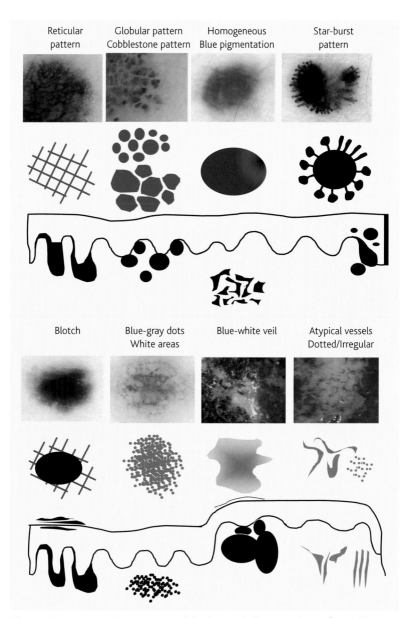

Figure 1.2 Dermoscopic structures and the histopathology correlation (see Table 1.1 for definitions)

Two-step dermoscopy algorithm

2

The two-step dermoscopy algorithm forms the foundation on which dermoscopic differential diagnosis is based upon (Figure 2.1).

First step

In the first step the dermoscopist needs to classify the lesion under investigation as melanocytic or non-melanocytic. This classification is based on certain structures that, when present, help to correctly classify the lesion as melanocytic (see Chapter 1 for definitions and examples of network, pseudonetwork, globules, streaks, homogeneous blue pigmentation and parallel pattern), basal cell carcinoma (BCC), hemangioma, seborrheic keratosis or dermatofibroma. If the lesion does not have any positive criteria for a melanocytic lesion and also lacks any positive criteria for a non-melanocytic lesion then the lesion needs to be considered, by default, to be of melanocytic origin (Figure 2.2). These so-called featureless melanocytic lesions need to be viewed with caution, since melanoma can present in this manner, especially in the presence, within the lesion, of irregular vessels and dotted vessels (see Chapter 3b on vascular structures).

Second step

If the lesion has criteria for a melanocytic lesion, the second step in the two-step dermoscopy algorithm can be applied. The second step helps to differentiate between benign nevi and melanoma. To this end, multiple algorithms have been created including "pattern analysis", "ABCD rule", "Menzies method" and the "7-point checklist" (see Chapters 4a– 4d).

Novice dermoscopists may find the ABCD rule, Menzies method and 7-point checklist most helpful. However, experienced dermoscopists almost exclusively rely on pattern recognition to help differentiate between benign nevi and melanoma.

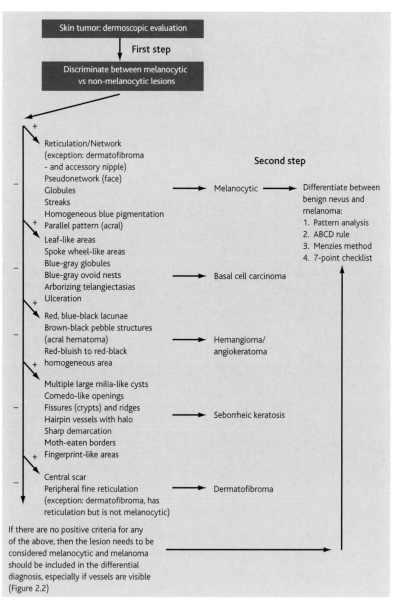

Figure 2.1 Two-step dermoscopy algorithm.

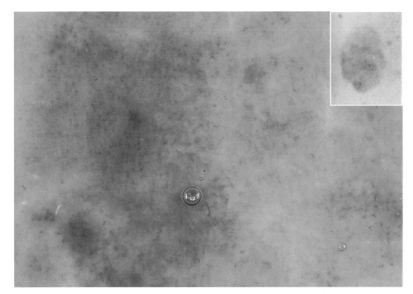

Figure 2.2 *This 0.85 mm invasive melanoma lacks any criteria for melanocytic neoplasm and also lacks features for non-melanocytic lesion. Thus, this lesion, by default, needs to be considered as a melanocytic tumor. Notice the irregular vessels under dermoscopy.*

3 Non-melanocytic lesions

3a: Seborrheic keratoses and lentigo

Seborrheic keratoses (Figures A21, A22)

Clinical criteria

Early seborrheic keratoses (SK) are light to dark brown macules with sharply demarcated borders. As the lesions progress, they transform into papules or plaques with a waxy or stuck-on appearance. Some of these lesions can resemble melanoma.

Dermoscopy

■ *Milia-like cysts*

Milia-like cysts are whitish or yellowish round structures, corresponding to intraepidermal keratin-filled cysts (Figure 3.1). They are mainly seen in seborrheic keratoses but some small milia-like cysts can also be seen in congenital melanocytic nevi and rarely in other melanocytic tumors.

■ *Comedo-like openings (crypts, pseudofollicular openings)*

Comedo-like openings (with "blackhead-like plugs") are roundish structures of brown to black color which are mainly seen in seborrheic keratosis or, in some rare cases, in papillomatous melanocytic nevi. They correspond histopathologically to keratin-filled invaginations of the epidermis.

■ *Fissures and ridges ("brain-like" or "cerebriform" appearance)*

Fissures are irregular linear keratin-filled depressions. They may also be seen in melanocytic nevi with congenital patterns and in some dermal melanocytic nevi. Multiple fissures might give a "brain-like

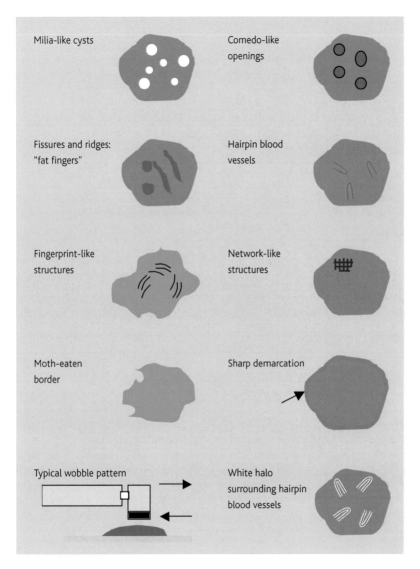

Milia-like cysts

Comedo-like openings

Fissures and ridges: "fat fingers"

Hairpin blood vessels

Fingerprint-like structures

Network-like structures

Moth-eaten border

Sharp demarcation

Typical wobble pattern

White halo surrounding hairpin blood vessels

Figure 3.1 Dermoscopy criteria of pigmented seborrheic keratoses.

appearance" to the lesion. This pattern has also been named "gyri and sulci" or "mountain and valley pattern". Hypo- or hyperpigmented gyri (ridges) have also been called "fat fingers".

■ *Fingerprint-like structures*

Some flat seborrheic keratoses (as well as solar lentigines) can show thin, brown, parallel lines resembling fingerprints.

■ *Moth-eaten border*

Some flat seborrheic keratosis (mainly on the face) have a concave border so that the pigment ends with a curved indentation which has been compared to a moth-eaten garment.

■ *Hairpin blood vessels ("typical")*

Hairpin blood vessels can be found in pigmented seborrheic keratosis. In most of the cases, clusters of hairpin blood vessels are grouped together, and each of them surrounded by a whitish halo, which gives them almost a "grape-like" appearance. They correspond to long capillary loops that are commonly seen in keratinizing tumors, and they are mainly found at the periphery of the lesions. Atypical hairpin blood vessels may be seen in thick melanomas.

■ *Network-like structures*

Pigmented seborrheic keratoses can have structures resembling a pigment network (reticulation). This "reticulation" is different from the classic pigment network and does not correspond to melanin pigment in keratinocytes or in melanocytes along the dermal–epidermal junction. For this reason, the term "network-like structures" has been proposed. The grids of these network-like structures are much larger than those seen in a typical pigment network, and the holes do not correspond to the tips of the dermal papillae. The network appears to be due to keratin-filled structures (fissures, comedo-like openings).

■ *Sharp demarcation*

Sharp demarcation (abrupt cut-off of pigmentation at the border) is present in almost 90% of SK.

■ *Wobble test*

During the dermoscopic examination of any skin lesion, the dermoscope has to be placed on the surface of the lesion. However, the device can still be moved slightly in the horizontal plane, parallel to the skin surface, thus adding a dynamic approach. Typically, raised lesions "stick" to the dermoscope face-plate and follow the movement of the plate. Hence, in papular lesions, the superficial part of the lesion "stays stuck" to the dermoscope face-plate which displaces it from the skin surrounding the papule, thus, creating the "wobble sign". Seborrheic keratoses were found to have a specific wobble pattern: the lesion follows the movement of the dermoscope face-plate, leaving back the surrounding skin, and the static image of the SK does not change because the stiff, papular component cannot be moved separately from the surface of the lesion itself. This sign reflects the consistency of the lesion, which is rather stiff and rigid compared to dermal nevi.

Solar lentigo (Figure A11)

Solar lentigines are formed due to increased accumulation of melanin in keratinocytes.

Clinical criteria

Solar lentigines may be oval, round or irregular in shape and can vary from a few millimeters to a few centimeters in diameter. Most lesions have a uniform light brown color. However, there are instances when they vary from dark brown to black. One variant of solar lentigo, "ink-spot" lentigo, has a jet-black color.

Dermoscopy

■ Moth-eaten border: A sharply demarcated and irregularly concave border resembling a moth-eaten garment is characteristic of solar lentigines.

■ A faint pigment network can be seen. The network corresponds to melanocytes and melanin-filled keratinocytes in the elongated rete ridges.

- "Fingerprint-like" structures.

- Structureless areas: Many lesions have no distinct dermoscopic structures. They appear as light brown structureless areas.

- Pseudonetwork: can frequently be found in lentigines located on the face and scalp.

Ink-spot lentigo

Dermoscopic criteria

- These lesions have a typical, prominent, black, thickened pigment network over the entire lesion. In some cases the network seems to have a three-dimensional appearance.

3b: Vascular lesions

Vascular lesions may be congenital or acquired and are often classified as either hemangiomas (e.g.strawberry hemangioma) or as vascular malformations (e.g. port-wine stain). The common dermoscopic feature in vascular lesions is the presence of "lacunae"(also called "saccules").

Cherry hemangiomas (Figures A23, A24)

Clinical aspect

Cherry hemangiomas are very common cutaneous tumors. Lesions are often widespread and are predominantly located on the trunk. Cherry hemangiomas have a variable appearance, ranging from small red macules to larger, dome-shaped, or polypoid papules. The colors of these lesions are typically bright cherry-red, but others may appear more violaceous. In some rare cases a partial thrombosis of the angioma appears clinically as a focal change of color, including black. This may clinically resemble melanoma. In addition, deeply red or violaceous nodular lesions may clinically mimic primary nodular melanoma or metastatic melanoma.

The diagnosis of cherry hemangiomas or other vascular lesions is generally made on clinical examination; however, dermoscopy may aid in their differentiation from melanomas in clinically suspicious lesions (Figure 3.2).

Dermoscopic criteria

■ Multiple, well-demarcated, red to blue-red or blue-black to maroon, round to oval structures called lacunae. Lacunae commonly vary in size and color within a given lesion and may be either tightly clustered or loosely scattered throughout. Often, lacunae are situated on a background of bluish-red pigmentation.

■ Absence of a pigmented network, globules and/or branched streaks.

■ Hemangiomas that develop a partial thrombosis can acquire a focal blue-black color and resemble melanomas.

15

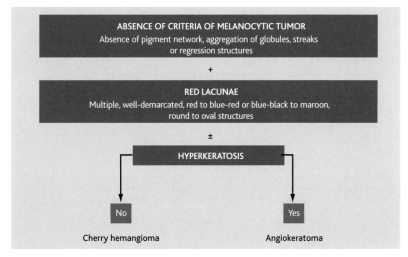

Figure 3.2 Simplified algorithm of the dermoscopic criteria of vascular tumors

Angiokeratomas (Figue A24)

Clinical criteria

Angiokeratomas are a group of unrelated, superficial, vascular ectasias that occur in conjunction with overlying hyperkeratosis.

Dermoscopic criteria

Solitary angiokeratomas vary in their dermoscopic appearance, depending on the lesion's age and on the presence or absence of thrombosis. The degree of hyperkeratosis increases as the lesion ages. Early lesions are dermoscopically indistinguishable from hemangiomas. The dermoscopic criteria are:

■ Absence of any criterion for a melanocytic lesion (pigmented network, globules or branched streaks).

■ The lacunae in angiokeratomas tend to be morphologically less well-defined than in cherry hemangiomas.

- Overlying whitish yellow hue, resulting from the increasingly acanthotic and hyperkeratotic epidermis, can be seen in some cases.

- In cases where the lesion is traumatized and/or thrombosed, angiokeratomas appear as previously described but with a focal crusted area of homogeneous, confluent blue-black pigment.

- In other cases, the entire lesion may become thrombosed, appearing as homogeneous, confluent, dark bluish-black pigment that is sharply demarcated at the periphery. Commonly, these lesions also have a prominent surrounding reddish halo. The etiology of the thrombosis is often trauma-induced.

If dermoscopic structures other than lacunae are seen, a diagnosis of something other than a benign vascular lesion should be strongly considered.

3c: Dermatofibroma (Figures A23, A25)

Dermatofibromas are common cutaneous tumors that can sometimes simulate atypical nevi or melanoma. On palpation, lesions are firm and they exhibit the characteristic tethering of the overlying epidermis to the underlying lesion, thus producing the "dimple sign" upon lateral compression.

By dermoscopy, dermatofibromas exhibit a "central white macule" (scar), consisting of a structureless area corresponding to the fibrotic area of the tumor. At the periphery of the lesion there is usually a tan to dark brown delicate pigment network formed by pigmentation of the basal layer. One can also observe ring-like globules that are formed from hyperpigmented and flattened rete ridges. Also one can see blood vessels in the center white macular area.

The dermoscopic criteria for the identification of dermatofibroma is given in Table 3.1.

Table 3.1 Dermoscopic criteria for dermatofibroma

Feature	Description
Central white patch	Central white scar-like macule. Reticulation, vessels and globule-like structures can be present in this area. In large lesions the central white macule can be replaced by central white reticulation
Peripheral thin reticulation	Delicate tan to dark brown or grayish reticulation at the periphery of the lesion. In some cases the brown pigmentation is diffuse and the reticulation cannot be seen

3d: Basal cell carcinoma (Figures A26–A29)

Dermoscopy is very useful in the identification of pigmented basal cell carcinoma (BCC) and in differentiating it from melanoma. The dermoscopic criteria for BCC include:

■ lack of features suggestive of a melanocytic lesion (Chapter 2)

■ presence of at least one positive feature for BCC listed in Table 3.2.

The dermoscopic criteria for the identification of BCC is given in Figure A26

Other features commonly seen in pigmented and non-pigmented BCC are shiny pink-white areas that are structureless. Non-pigmented BCC often have an erythematous blush surrounding the lesion and also have arborizing telangiectasia.

Negative feature (cannot be found):

Absence of pigment network

Positive features (at least one of the following must be present):

Large gray-blue ovoid nests
Confluent or near-confluent pigmented ovoid or elongated areas, larger than globules, and not visibly connected to the main pigmented tumor body

Multiple blue-gray globules
Blue-gray globules are multiple round blue-grayish structures that are larger than blue dots of "peppering"

Maple leaf-like areas
Brown to gray-blue discrete bulbous extensions forming a leaf-like pattern. They never arise from a pigment network and usually do not arise from an adjacent confluent pigmented area

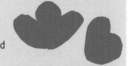

Spokewheel areas
Radial projections, usually tan but sometimes blue or gray, meeting at a darker central axel or hub

Arborizing "tree-like" telangiectasia
Thick and arborizing vessels on the surface of the tumor

Ulceration
Denuded area of skin, often covered by a serosanguineous crust. In superficial BCC, it is common to see multiple ulcers, most of which are located at the periphery of the lesion and often covered by black sanguineous crusts

Table 3.2 Dermoscopic criteria for BCC

Melanocytic algorithms

4a: Pattern analysis

Melanocytic tumors may display one or more of the structures (for definitions see Chapter 1) shown in Box 4.1.

Melanocytic tumors may display one or more of the following colors: light brown, dark brown, gray, black, red, white and blue. The location and distribution of the below-mentioned structures (Box 4.1) and colors form distinct global "patterns" that are characteristic of certain specific lesions. In general, benign lesions have dermoscopic structures and colors distributed symmetrically and melanomas have them distributed asymmetrically (A36, A37). In addition to the global patterns there are local features that may prove to be of significance (Table 4.2).

The term "multicomponent" pattern means that the lesion has three or more structures. See Chapter 1 for definitions of structures. Lesions with a multicomponent pattern or any lesion displaying local structures as outlined in Table 4.2 should be viewed with caution.

Box 4.1 Structures of melanocytic tumors

1. Network, pseudonetwork, parallel pattern and negative network (reverse pigment network)
2. Streaks (radial streaming, pseudopods)
3. Branched streaks
4. Dots
5. Globules
6. Cobblestone globules
7. Blotches
8. Hypopigmented/depigmented (structureless) areas
9. Blue-white veil
10. Regression structures ("peppering")
11. Vascular (milky-red areas, vessels)

The global patterns for melanocytic lesions are given in Table 4.1

Table 4.1 *Global patterns for melanocytic lesions*

Global pattern	Definition	Benign vs malignant
Reticular	Lesion composed almost entirely of a pigment network *Typical pigment network* Atypical pigment network 	In benign lesions, the pigment network is regular and delicate, with regular circular to oval, thin-lined meshes that thin out at the periphery (typical pigment network). The distribution of this relatively homogeneous typical network is usually symmetric. The network can be present as an uninterrupted mesh throughout the lesion or can be present throughout the lesion in a patchy pattern (patchy network pattern) In melanoma and many dysplastic nevi the network is often prominent, irregular, with variable mesh size and configuration that has an abrupt cut off at the periphery (atypical pigment network). The distribution of this heterogeneous atypical network is usually asymmetric
Globular	Lesion composed almost entirely of round to oval globules *Typical globular pattern* 	In benign lesions, the globules are regular and uniform in size, distributed symmetrically and homogeneously throughout the lesion and are brown in color

Table 4.1 Continued

Global pattern	Definition	Benign vs malignant
Globular	*Atypical globular pattern* 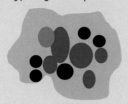	In melanoma and some dysplastic nevi, the globules are of different sizes and haphazardly spaced (irregular) and unevenly distributed. Globules with a reddish color are highly suggestive of melanoma
Cobblestone	Lesion composed of closely aggregated, large, angulated globules resembling cobblestones. This pattern can be considered as a variant of the globular pattern *Cobblestone pattern*	In benign lesions, the cobblestone globules are symmetrically distributed throughout the lesion. This pattern is frequently seen in congenital nevi. In melanoma, the cobblestone globules are not uniform and often have a reddish color. Other structures such as regression structures and polymorphous vascular structures are also frequently seen
Reticulo-globular	Lesion composed of both network and globules 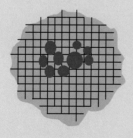	In benign lesions, the distribution of the network and globules is symmetric. Lesions will often have centrally placed globules and peripherally placed fine reticulation (this pattern is commonly seen in congenital nevi). Enlarging nevi can have central reticulation, with a rim of globules at the periphery. In melanoma and some dysplastic nevi, the distribution of the network and globules is asymmetric. The network is often atypical and the globules are usually irregular in size, shape and color

Table 4.1 Continued

Global pattern	Definition	Benign vs malignant
Homogeneous	Lesion with diffuse, brown, gray-blue to gray-black or reddish black pigmentation without pigment network or any other discernible structures (structureless) 	In benign nevi, the homogeneous pattern is usually brown in color. However, blue nevi tend to have a "steel" blue homogeneous color throughout. In melanoma, the homogeneous pattern is usually seen in association with fine vascular structures
Reticulo-homogeneous	Lesions with a network located at the periphery. The center of the lesion can have a symmetric area of hypopigmentation or a central area with a structureless blotch 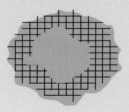	This type of pattern is often seen in dysplastic nevi. It is not uncommon to also see a few black dots in such lesions. The entire lesion is symmetric. In the presence of black dots, such a lesion would be classified as a multicomponent pattern. In melanoma, the distribution of the hypopigmented area or hyperpigmented blotch will be asymmetric and will often be found at the periphery of the lesion, as opposed to the center.

Table 4.1 Continued

Global pattern	Definition	Benign vs malignant
Starburst	Lesions with pigmented streaks or globules that are in a radial arrangement around the periphery of a lesion	In benign nevi, the radial arrangement of streaks or globules is symmetric and is present around the entire periphery of the lesion. This pattern is commonly seen in Spitz nevi and Reed nevi.

Typical starburst pattern

Atypical starburst pattern

In melanoma the periphery may have both streaks and globules. These structures are almost never seen encompassing the entire periphery

| Parallel | Lesion with parallel pigmented lines. This pattern is exclusively found in melanocytic lesions on palms and soles | In benign nevi the parallel lines tend to be thin and homogeneous. The pigment is found in the sulcus superficialis and forms the parallel furrow pattern |

Parallel furrow pattern

Table 4.1 Continued

Global pattern	Definition	Benign vs malignant
Parallel	*Parallel ridge pattern*	In melanoma, the parallel lines tend to be thick and heterogeneous. The pigment is found in the crest, and thus the openings of the eccrine ducts can often be seen in the center of the pigmented lines. This pattern is called the parallel ridge pattern
Multi component	Three or more distinct structures (Box 4.1) within the same lesion	In benign nevi, the individual structures tend to be homogeneous and the structures are distributed in a symmetric manner. For example, a lesion may have central globules, peripheral reticulation and symmetrically distributed dots. Most nevi with a multicomponent pattern are either congenital or dysplastic. In melanoma the individual structures tend to be atypical/irregular and the structures are distributed asymmetrically
Non-specific	Lesion that does not fit one of the above-mentioned patterns	This pattern does not have any diagnostic implications. However, if vessels (especially when dotted or irregular linear) are seen, then melanoma should be strongly considered in the differential

Besides the global patterns described above it is important to remember the significance of the structures shown in Table 4.2.

Table 4.2 Local features for melanocytic lesions

Structure	Benign	Melanoma and some dysplastic nevi
Streaks (radial streaming or pseudopods)	Present uniformly around the entire lesion. Such a lesion would be classified as having a "starburst" pattern	Present focally and asymmetrically distributed at the periphery
Dots/Globules	Dots and globules of regular size, shape and distribution may be found in the center of benign nevi (junctional). They are often found directly overlying the lines of the network	Irregularly distributed dots and globules of varying sizes and shapes can be seen centrally and at the periphery of the lesion and often are found off the network
Blue-whitish veil	A confluent, bluish-whitish pigmentation can be seen focally in the center of some benign nevi	It is frequently found in melanomas overlying areas of regression. It is often present asymmetrically distributed or can cover almost the entire lesion
Regression structures (white scar-like areas and blue-gray peppering)	Associated with fibrosis and melanosis. In benign nevi regression, structures are usually mild (less than 25% of the entire lesion)	These structures are commonly seen in the areas of melanoma with a thin Breslow depth

Table 4.2 Continued

Structure	Benign	Melanoma and some dysplastic nevi
Blotches	Blotches are focal hyperpigmented (black) areas that obscure underlying structures and comprise at least 10% of the lesion area. They can occur centrally or throughout the entire lesion in benign nevi. One solitary blotch is the norm for benign nevi	Blotches in melanoma tend to be located peripherally and frequently are multiple
Hypopigmented areas (structureless/ homogeneous)	Hypopigmented areas are focal areas devoid of structures, lightly pigmented, and comprise at least 10% of the lesion area. These areas can be seen in dysplastic nevi and tend to be located centrally	Hypopigmented areas in melanomas tend to be located at the periphery.
Vascular patterns	Vascular structures include hairpin, dotted, linear-irregular, torturous/cork-screw, comma-shaped, crown, glomerular and arborizing. The presence of comma vessels is suggestive of an intradermal nevus	The presence of vessels other than comma vessels is suggestive of an irritated nevus or melanoma

NB Atypical pigment network and reverse pigment network are seen in melanomas and dysplastic nevi.

Patterns seen in non-melanocytic lesions are shown in Table 4.3.

Table 4.3 Structural patterns for non-melanocytic lesions

Pattern	Definition	Lesion
Lacunae or saccules	Red, blue or black lacunae distributed homogeneously throughout the lesion	Angiomas, hemangiomas, vascular malformations, angiokeratomas. In these vascular lesions no structures other than lacuna are present. However, bluish-white veil and scar-like areas may be seen
Cerebriform or fissured	Thick furrows and ridges (cerebriform pattern) with a sharp demarcation	Seborrheic keratosis. Other structures commonly seen in SK include moth-eaten border, fingerprint-like structures, milia-like- cysts, comedo-like openings and regular hairpin vessels surrounded by hypopigmented halo
Central scar with peripheral fine network	Centrally placed hypopigmented scar that is often stellate. The periphery is composed of a fine network. Donut-shaped, globule-like structures are frequently seen in the center of the lesion	Dermatofibroma
Multiple structures including arborizing vessels, leaf-like areas or spokewheel-like areas	Presence of arborizing vessels, leaf-like areas, spokewheel-like structures, large blue-gray ovoid nests, multiple blue-gray globules and ulceration	Basal cell carcinoma

Vascular patterns in tumoral lesions are given in Table 4.4.

Table 4.4 Vascular patterns in tumoral lesions

Pattern	Correlation	
Red lagoons	Sharply demarcated globular structures Colors: red, violaceous, brownish, bluish or black Absence of vessels or other pigmented structures inside the lagoons Significance: hemangiomas or angiokeratomas	
Hairpin vessels	Elongated vessels resembling hairpins Significance: when fine and surrounded by hypopigmented halo, seborrheic heratosis and other keratonizing tumors Irregular and thick: melanoma, Spitz nevus	
Irregular polymorphous vessels	Multiple vessels with different shapes inlcuding comma, dotted irregular lines, cork-screw, glomerular and others Significance: melanoma	
Dotted vessels	Small vessels resembling the head of a pin. Significance: vertical vessels seen in Spitz nevus or melanoma. Can also be seen in other lesions such as psoriasis and squamous cell carcinoma	

Table 4.4 Continued

Pattern	Correlation	
Comma-like vessels	Resembling the shape of a comma Significance: compound or dermal nevus	
Clusters of "glomerular" vessels	Small and fine coiled vessels Significance: Bowen's disease. Can also be seen in melanoma and in stasis dermatitis	
String of pearls	Globular vessels following a serpiginous distribution Significance: clear-cell acanthoma	
Crown vessels	Radial wreath-like or individual vessels at the periphery of the tumor. White-yellow globules, they can be seen in the center of the tumor Significance: sebaceous gland hyperplasia	
Corkscrew vessels	Irregular and thick coiled vessels Significance: melanoma including metastasis	
Arborizing vessels	Resembling the branches of a tree Significance: basal cell carcinoma	

4b: ABCD rule of dermoscopy

This second-step algorithm (see Chapter 2) is based on a scoring system for melanocytic neoplasms that differentiates them into benign, suspicious and malignant categories. This is accomplished by calculating a total dermoscopy score (TDS) for the lesion. The scores are divided into three groups as shown in Table 4.5.

Table 4.5 Scoring system for melanocytic neoplasms

Category	Score range
Benign	< 4.75
Suspicious	4.75 to 5.45
Malignant	> 5.45

The distribution of scores is shown in Figure 4.1.

Other features of the ABCD rule of dermoscopy are detailed in Tables 4.6 and 4.7, Figure 4.2 and Box 4.2.

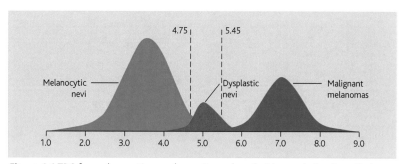

Figure 4.1 TDS for melanocytic neoplasms. Reproduced with permission from Stolz, Braun–Falco, Bilek et al, Colour atlas of dermatoscopy, 2nd edn. Berlin: Blackwell; 2002.

Table 4.6 Definition of the ABCD acronym

Dermoscopic features	Definition
A = Asymmetry	The lesion is bisected by two lines that are placed 90° to each other. The first line attempts to bisect the lesion at the division of "most symmetry" and the other line is then placed 90° to it. Symmetry takes into account the contour, colors and structures within a lesion. Lesions that are symmetric in both axes are given zero points, one axis asymmetry 1 point and biaxial asymmetry 2 points. Thus, the points range from 0 to 2
B = Border sharpness	First, the lesion is divided into eight equal pie-shaped pieces. Next, one counts the number of segments that have an abrupt perimeter cutoff. Thus, the points range from 0 to 8
C = Colors	Number of the following colors present: light brown, dark brown, black, red, white, blue-gray. Thus, the points range from 1 to 6
D = Dermoscopic structures	Number of following 5 structures: dots, globules, structureless (homogeneous) areas, network and branched streaks. Thus, the points range from 1 to 5

NB Structureless areas can be either hypopigmented or hyperpigmented (blotch). Branched streaks include streaks, pseudopods, radial streaming and branched streaks, as defined in Chapter 1.

Table 4.7 Calculation of the total dermoscopy score (TDS)

Feature	Points	Weight factor	TDS score
Asymmetry	0–2	× 1.3	0–2.6
Border sharpness	0–8	× 0.1	0–0.8
Colors	1–6	× 0.5	0.5–3.0
Dermoscopic structures	1–5	× 0.5	0.5–2.5
Total dermoscopy score (TDS range)			1.0–8.9

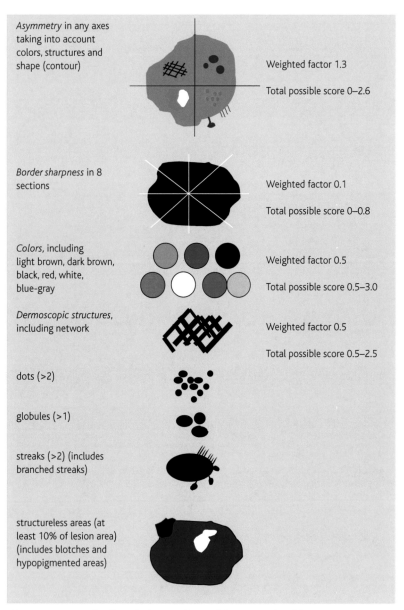

Asymmetry in any axes taking into account colors, structures and shape (contour)

Weighted factor 1.3

Total possible score 0–2.6

Border sharpness in 8 sections

Weighted factor 0.1

Total possible score 0–0.8

Colors, including light brown, dark brown, black, red, white, blue-gray

Weighted factor 0.5

Total possible score 0.5–3.0

Dermoscopic structures, including network

Weighted factor 0.5

Total possible score 0.5–2.5

dots (>2)

globules (>1)

streaks (>2) (includes branched streaks)

structureless areas (at least 10% of lesion area) (includes blotches and hypopigmented areas)

Figure 4.2 Criteria for the calculation of TDS of the ABCD rule of dermoscopy

Box 4.2 *Notes concerning the ABCD rule of dermoscopy*

1. Certain melanocytic nevi are diagnosed dermoscopically by "Gestalt" (overall impression) and not by the ABCD dermoscopy scoring system:
   - blue nevus
   - intradermal nevus (globular; papillomatous)
   - Spitz/Reed nevus
   - congenital nevus
   - recurrent nevus
   - nevus spilus

2. Additional dermoscopic clues:
   Clues for melanoma not included in the ABCD dermoscopy scoring system include:
   - melanin peppering (regression structures)
   - vessels (dot-like; irregular linear)
   - red dots/globules
   - milky-red areas

3. Indeterminate lesions:
   - indeterminate dermoscopic patterns can be seen in both benign and malignant melanocytic neoplasms
   - the ABCD rule fails in the detection of some early small malignant melanomas because these lesions can be symmetric. Thus, such lesions cannot be dermoscopically differentiated by this method

4. Featureless melanomas:
   - Clinically and dermoscopically they lack melanoma-specific features. They also lack features and patterns of benign lesions
   - Clue: dermoscopically atypical vascular patterns (dotted and irregular linear) in a pink lesion
   - LOOK FOR PIGMENTED REMNANTS!

4c: Seven-point checklist

The seven-point checklist is a simplification of pattern analysis. A melanocytic lesion is evaluated for the presence of three major criteria (each with a weighted factor of 2) and four minor criteria (each with a weighted factor of 1).

Major criteria (each assigned a score of 2)

1. Atypical pigment network

The term "atypical" pigment network defines a black, brown or gray network with irregular holes and thick lines. An atypical network is usually found in focal areas within the lesion.

2. Blue-white veil

Dermoscopically, this feature appears as an irregular, structureless area of confluent blue pigmentation with an overlying white "ground-glass" film. The pigmentation should not occupy the entire lesion; it usually corresponds to a clinically elevated portion of the lesion, and corresponds to melanin in the deep dermis. It must be differentiated from gray-blue areas (blue pepper-like granules, multiple blue-gray dots) that are commonly associated with white scar-like depigmentation in areas of regression, which are usually found in the thin areas of melanomas.

3. Atypical vascular pattern

A vascular pattern may be observed in melanomas undergoing regression but also in hypopigmented or amelanotic melanomas. The following morphologic variations of atypical vascular pattern can be distinguished:

- linear-irregular vessels, which are presumably the expression of neovascularization in a melanoma

- dotted vessels, which are vessels that are perpendicular to the skin surface

Minor criteria (each assigned a score of 1)

1. Irregular streaks (irregularly distributed)

Radial streaming and pseudopods (irregular extensions) are considered as a single criterion in the seven-point checklist. This is because, although morphologically dissimilar, they are both histopathologically correlated with confluent radial junctional nests of melanocytes. To be scored, streaks must be irregularly distributed at the edge of the lesion.

2. Dots/globules (irregularly distributed)

These dermoscopic structures are also considered as a single criterion in the seven-point checklist. Although dots and globules are distinguished by their size, both may be black or brown. To be scored, dots/globules must be irregularly distributed within the lesion.

3. Blotches (irregularly distributed)

These are black, brown and/or gray structureless areas, asymmetrically and irregularly distributed within the lesion.

4. Regression structures

On the basis of their similar histopathologic significance, white (scar-like) depigmentation and gray-blue areas (blue pepper-like granules) are included as a single criterion called "regression structures", the former being related to the presence of fibrosis and the latter to melanophages.

Interpretation

By a simple addition of the individual scores, a total score of 3 or more allows classification of the lesion as a melanoma, with a sensitivity of 95% and a specificity of 75% (Figure 4.3).

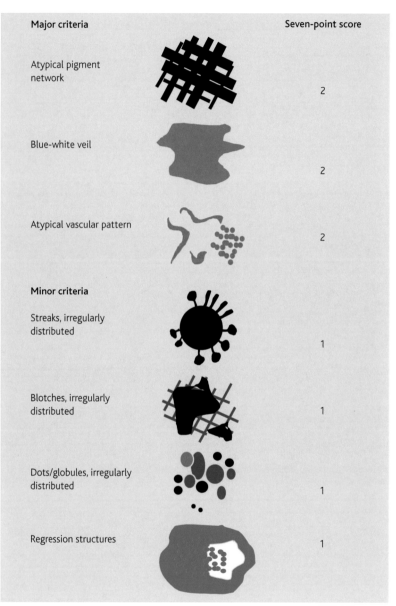

Major criteria		Seven-point score
Atypical pigment network		2
Blue-white veil		2
Atypical vascular pattern		2
Minor criteria		
Streaks, irregularly distributed		1
Blotches, irregularly distributed		1
Dots/globules, irregularly distributed		1
Regression structures		1

Figure 4.3 Seven-point checklist.

4d: Menzies method

This algorithm helps differentiate melanoma from melanocytic nevi. For a melanoma to be diagnosed, it must have *neither* of the two morphologic negative features *and* at least one or more of the nine positive features. The criteria used comprise the following negative and positive features (Figure 4.4).

Negative features – both features must be absent

■ **Symmetry of pattern**

This is symmetry of all dermoscopic structures, including color, along any axis through the center (of gravity) of the lesion. It does *not* require symmetry of shape. The presence of symmetry of the pigmentation pattern is often the immediate defining feature of benign pigmented lesions.

■ **Single color**

The colors scored are black, gray, blue, red, dark brown and tan. White is not scored. A single color excludes the diagnosis of melanoma. This is because malignant melanocytes often retain cellular melanin. Therefore, in melanoma, melanin occupies varied depths in the skin: from the stratum corneum, where it is seen as black; the mid-epidermis, as dark brown (often found in melanoma secondary to pagetoid invasion of the epidermis); the dermoepidermal junction, as tan; the upper dermis, as gray; and the mid-dermis, as blue.

In summary, most melanomas are asymmetric and have more than one color.

Positive features – at least one feature must be found to suspect melanoma

■ **Blue–white veil**

This is an irregular confluent blue pigmentation with an overlying "ground glass" white film or "veil". It cannot be associated with red-

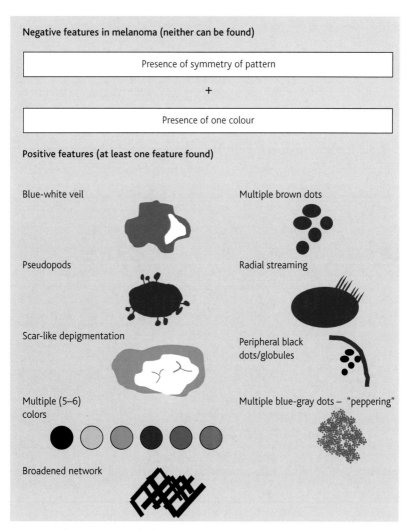

Negative features in melanoma (neither can be found)

Presence of symmetry of pattern

+

Presence of one colour

Positive features (at least one feature found)

Blue-white veil

Multiple brown dots

Pseudopods

Radial streaming

Scar-like depigmentation

Peripheral black dots/globules

Multiple (5–6) colors

Multiple blue-gray dots – "peppering"

Broadened network

Figure 4.4 The Menzies' method

blue lacunae found in hemangiomas or well-defined structures such as large ovoid nests seen in pigmented basal cell carcinomas. It can never occupy the entire lesion, as occurs with many blue nevi.

■ Multiple brown dots

These are focal aggregations of cells which histopathologically represent intraepidermal (suprabasal) melanoma cells. They should be distinguished by their small size (dots rather than globules) and should be multiple and focal rather than scattered sparsely.

■ Streaks

These are finger-like projections at the edge of the lesion, which may be linear extensions of an existing network but more often arise from the solid tumor. Histologically, they represent confluent radial nests of melanoma cells at the level of the dermoepidermal junction. Streaks are often seen in superficial spreading melanomas.

■ Pseudopods

These are similar to streaks except that they have bulbous "foot-like" enlargements at the end of the projections. They can arise from a pigmented network or from the solid pigmented border. They have the same histologic correlate as radial streaming. Pseudopods should never occupy a uniform circumferential position in melanoma, but they can in Spitz nevi.

■ Scar-like depigmentation

The chronic phase of regression may be seen as scarring. Scar-like depigmentations are seen as pure white, well-defined, irregular areas and should be distinguished from hypomelanotic areas commonly seen in benign nevi.

■ Peripheral black dots/globules

These are found at the periphery of a lesion. They are black in color in contrast to brown dots/globules commonly found in benign lesions. They have to be distinguished from central black dots/globules, which are found in some dysplastic nevi and some congenital melanocytic nevi.

■ Multiple (five to six) colors

In invasive melanoma, melanin is often found in multiple layers of the skin, from the stratum corneum to the mid-dermis. This, and the presence of increased vasculature, can lead to the presence of multiple colors. To be a significant "positive" feature there must be at least five colors from a possible total of six (red, tan, dark brown, black, gray and blue).

■ Multiple blue-gray dots ("peppering")

In areas of regression of melanocytic lesions, multiple blue-gray dots representing free melanin granules and melanin-laden macrophages (melanophages) can be found in the dermis. These are seen as partly aggregated blue-gray dots often described as "pepper-like" in morphology. When abundant, dermal melanin of regression structures may form blue homogeneous areas indistinguishable from blue-white veil.

Multiple blue-gray dots are also a common feature of lentigo maligna (in-situ melanoma) and lichen-planus-like keratosis.

■ Broadened network

This is an increase in the width of the "grids" (also called "cords" or "lines") of the pigmented net found in melanocytic lesions. This broadening of the network is usually found focally in melanoma, rather than uniformly throughout the lesion. Broadened network (called pseudonetwork) is also a common feature of facial lentigo maligna.

4e: Three-point checklist

The three-point checklist is based on a simplified pattern analysis and is intended for use by non-experts as a screening technique. The three-point checklist does not differentiate between melanocytic and non-melanocytic lesions. Its aim is to identify all potentially malignant lesions, including basal cell carcinoma and melanoma, with a high degree of sensitivity. Remarkably, the sensitivity for detecting malignancy by non-experts using the three-point checklist has reached 96.3%, however, as is true for all screening techniques, the specificity achieved by non-experts was much lower (32.8%) than by experts (94.2%).

The three-point checklist requires the examiner to assess the lesion for only three dermoscopic criteria: (1) asymmetry, (2) atypical network and (3) blue-white structures. The presence of two or three features suggests that the lesion under investigation is suspect for malignancy (Figure 4.5).

Asymmetry in any axes taking into account colors and structures but not shape

Symmetry in structures

Asymmetry in structures

Atypical network considered when the lines of the net have differences in thickness and the sizes of the holes are non-homogeneous. The atypical network is usually irregularly distributed within the lesion

*Blue-white structures** include any white and/or any blue color present in the lesions

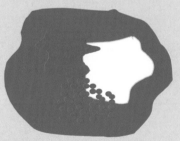

*Blue-white structures include peppering (corresponding to melanophages); blue-white veil (orthokeratotic hyperkeratosis overlying a pigmented tumor); whitish scar (fibrosis); or blue structures, as seen in basal cell carcinoma (e.g. blue-gray ovoid nests, blue-gray globules).

Figure 4.5 *Criteria of the three-point checklist*

5 Melanocytic lesions

5a: Melanocytic nevi

Melanocytic nevi include a broad spectrum of benign neoplasms derived from melanocytes. These lesions have a marked variability in their clinical and dermoscopic characteristics. An outline of the global patterns and local structures is presented in Chapters 1 and 4a.

- Common melanocytic nevi:
  - junctional
  - compound
  - dermal

- Blue nevus and combined nevus

- Dysplastic nevus

- Spitz nevus

- Congenital nevus

- Recurrent nevus

Junctional nevi

- On dermoscopy, these macular lesions usually appear as a light brown or darker brown network. The thickness of the lines is relatively uniform and the holes of the network vary little in area or shape.

- The margins fade gradually at the periphery of the lesion.

- At times, black dots (usually superimposed on the network lines) and brown globules can be seen (often at the center or encircling the periphery of the lesion).

Compound melanocytic nevi

■ These lesions are usually raised (slightly elevated to polypoid) and can show various combinations of network, globules, dots and structureless (homogeneous) areas.

■ Colors are usually various shades of light brown and dark brown.

■ The edges of such lesions tend to be rather regular and fade gradually into the surrounding skin.

Intradermal melanocytic nevi

■ These lesions are elevated (dome-shaped; sessile to polypoid) and have a sparse to absent network and globular pattern.

■ Cerebriform intradermal nevi have gyri and sulci and can have varying degrees of pigmentation (most often light brown, dark brown or gray-blue); they are sometimes amelanotic.

■ Occasionally, small and sparse milia-like cysts and comedo-like structures are seen.

■ Comma-like blood vessels are frequently found.

■ Generally, lesions are round or oval in shape.

■ Sometimes, a few extra hairs emerge from the surface of such nevi.

Blue nevi (Figure A13)

■ Well-circumscribed, homogeneous, relatively confluent blue-gray to blue-black pigmented lesions (Figure A13). The prototypic blue nevus is usually round or oval, slightly elevated and palpable, with a uniform steel-blue color throughout the lesion. At times, there is a diffuse blue-white veil-like appearance on its entire surface.

■ Absence of a network, dots/globules, branched streaks, vessels, regression and/or additional colors. The presence of any of these additional structures should alert one to the possibility of nodular primary or metastatic melanomas which, on occasion, may dermoscopically mimic blue nevi.

- Blue nevi can undergo focal fibrosis, causing mottled white scar-like areas within the lesion.

- Blue nevi tend to gradually fade in color into the surrounding skin.

Combined nevi

Definition

A combined nevus is composed of two or more distinct cell populations, which are usually reflected clinically by different colors and more clearly demonstrated by visualization with the dermoscope.

Because of their multicolored appearance on visual inspection, combined nevi are often clinically suspicious for melanomas. However, dermoscopy can sometimes aid in their differentiation.

Dermoscopic criteria

- Combined nevi can present with a multicomponent pattern that reflects the combination of their constituent cellular components. Thus, a typical pigment network reflecting the junctional melanocytic nevus component appears juxtaposed to a discrete area of homogeneous blue-gray pigmentation, reflecting the blue nevus component. If the pigmented network itself is irregular or if the lesion has any other additional features of melanoma – such as irregular dots/globules, blood vessels, streaks (pseudopods), branched streaks, regression, multiple colors – then the lesion should be biopsied to rule out melanoma.

- The homogeneous, confluent blue-gray pigmentation may occur either focally or extend throughout the entire lesion.

- Finally, the reverse pattern may also occur: a focal area of regular, pigmented network juxtaposed within the homogeneous, confluent, blue-gray pigmentation.

Dysplastic nevi

Definition

Clinically, dysplastic nevi (DN) are atypical moles which share some or all of the ABCD (A = Asymmetry; B = Border irregularity; C = Color variability; D = Diameter greater than 6 mm) of malignant melanoma (MM).

Dermoscopic criteria

Dermoscopically, there is a very broad spectrum of dysplastic nevi which can be classified into two groups as follows:

"Benign" pattern dysplastic nevi

Despite their clinical features, which share the ABCDs of MM, most DN on dermoscopic examination can be readily identified as having benign patterns. Thus, by dermoscopy, these lesions can have appearances seen in common melanocytic nevi. Often, however, the patterns, colors and structures are relatively ordered. Structureless (homogeneous) areas are more frequently observed than in common melanocytic nevi. Dots, globules, black blotches, network, vascular patterns and colors can vary greatly within the lesion. Segments of the margin of DN can be abrupt. Generally, DN lose some or all of the architectural order (symmetry, uniformity, sparseness of colors) seen in common melanocytic nevi. Compared with common melanocytic nevi, which are usually less than 6 mm in diameter, it is not exceptional for DN to be 10–15 mm or more in largest diameter. An important diagnostic clue in the differential diagnosis of congenital melanocytic nevi and DN is the lack of hypertrichosis and the usual lack of a blue hue in DN.

There are five patterns (Figure A36) found invariably to be benign in patients who have the classic atypical mole syndrome (i.e., patients who have the triad of 100 or more melanocytic nevi, at least one nevus 8 mm or larger in diameter and at least one dysplastic nevus). These patterns are:

- diffuse network pattern

- patchy network pattern

- peripheral network pattern with central hypopigmentation pattern

- peripheral network pattern with central hyperpigmentation

- peripheral network pattern with central uniform globules.

In each of these five patterns, the network must be uniform and fade at the perimeter of the lesion.

The implication of classifying a DN as "indeterminate" is that it is not possible dermoscopically to differentiate the lesion from melanoma. "Indeterminate" DN have a very broad spectrum of dermoscopic atypicalities. At one end of this spectrum are slightly atypical nevi that have some minor, potentially disconcerting, features that might lead to closer follow-up or sequential dermoscopic imaging. At the other end of the spectrum, it is impossible dermoscopically to differentiate DN from early melanoma. Although rare, white scar-like depigmentation, streaks/pseudopods, blue-white veil, regression with peppering, and five or more colors (tan, dark brown, black, gray, blue and red) can be seen.

Spitz and Reed nevi (Figure A3)

Spitz nevi can appear as reddish to brownish skin tumors. Reed nevi are mostly dark brown to black in color. Specific dermoscopic features can be found in both Spitz and Reed nevi. However, there are instances in which both dermoscopy and histopathology cannot conclusively differentiate between Spitz/Reed nevi and cutaneous melanoma.

A variety of dermoscopic patterns is described for Spitz/Reed nevi (Figure 5.1). This classification is helpful in the dermoscopic diagnosis, but in some cases the differentiation from a cutaneous melanoma is impossible.

Globular pattern

Symmetric globular pattern with brown globules or dots. Large symmetric globules can often be observed at the periphery of the lesion, forming a starburst-like pattern. In the center of the lesion, symmetric gray-blue colors can be found and occasionally dotted vessels may also be seen. Some Spitz nevi can have large globules distributed through the lesion.

Starburst pattern

All around the periphery, one observes circumferentially distributed streaks, pseudopods or globules. This arrangement has been compared to the image of an exploding star. In some lesions, only a portion of the peripheral rim will have the starburst pattern, making the differential diagnosis of melanoma difficult.

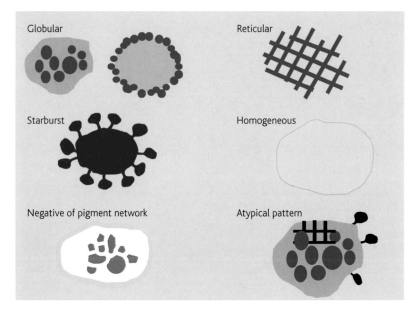

Figure 5.1 Dermoscopic patterns of Spitz and Reed nevi.

Reticular pattern

A prominent thickened dark brown to black network can be found.

Homogeneous pattern

Homogeneous light brown to reddish pigmentation without any structures can be observed. In the case of a reddish homogeneous tumor with or without visible vessels, the possibility of melanoma must be entertained and excluded.

Atypical pattern

Some Spitz and Reed nevi have the typical dermoscopic features of melanoma, consisting of asymmetry and different colors with black, brown, gray to blue pigmentation. Also, different structures, such as prominent focal network areas, globules, homogeneous areas and streaks, can be found. Furthermore, pinpoint vessels can be seen. In the presence of these atypical features, it is not possible to differentiate between a benign and malignant skin tumor by dermoscopy. In these cases the final diagnosis will have to rest with histopathology. Lastly, some Spitz nevi can reveal a negative network pattern with light areas making up the grids of the network and dark areas filling the "holes".

Congenital nevus

Most small and medium congenital melanocytic nevus (CMN) are fairly homogeneous both clinically and dermoscopically. Large CMN are often heterogeneous, displaying multiple islands of color and irregular topography. However, each "island" within the large CMN tends to be fairly homogeneous in its appearance. Knowledge of the dermoscopic features and patterns common to CMN can aid physicians in following these lesions and recognizing aberrancy that may be suggestive of melanoma. In other words, if a change occurs or the dermoscopic pattern does not conform to the known CMN patterns, then a biopsy or an excision may be warranted.

Dermoscopic features of CMN

Dermoscopic evaluation of a CMN begins with the observation of dermoscopic structures (Table 5.1).

Other dermoscopic features seen in CMN

Other structures frequently observed in CMN viewed under dermoscopy are given in Table 5.2.

Dermoscopic patterns (Figure A36 and schematics)

After identifying the local dermoscopic features commonly seen in CMN, it becomes apparent that these nevi often form specific dermoscopic patterns (Table 5.3).

Table 5.1 Dermoscopic structures commonly observed in CMN

Pattern	Definition	Characteristics
Reticular network	Honeycomb-like network of brown-black pigment	Quality • Fine • Thick Distribution • Homogeneous throughout • Patchy throughout • Peripheral Specific type • Linear fragments (hyphal-like/branched streaks)
Globules	Sharply circumscribed, round to oval aggregates of brown-black pigment	Quality • Small • Large Distribution • Diffusely throughout (sparse or dense concentration) • Central Specific type • Cobblestone • Target
Diffuse background pigmentation	Diffuse distribution of brown background pigment	Overall structureless but some remnant structures may be seen • Reticular network fragments • Few globules

Conclusion

Dermoscopy has the potential to be enormously valuable in the diagnosis and follow-up of CMN. The classification system proposed in this chapter should provide the foundation for the recognition of CMN. Those CMN that do not conform to the known patterns described above should be viewed with caution. In addition, CMN with a multicomponent pattern should be followed closely or excised prophylactically.

Table 5.2 Other dermoscopic features seen in CMN

Feature	Definition
Milia-like cysts	White to yellow, rounded, often hazy structures resembling the small seeds or millets of various grain grasses
Hypertrichosis	Increased number of thicker hairs
Perifollicular pigment changes	Hypopigmentation or hyperpigmentation occurring around the hair follicles

Table 5.3 CMN dermoscopic patterns

Global pattern	Definition
Reticular	Primarily reticular in pattern
Globular	Primarily globular in pattern
Reticulo-globular	Peripheral reticulation in conjunction with central globules (symmetric)
Diffuse brown pigmentation	Primarily diffuse structureless pattern with or without reticular network fragments and/or remnant globules
Multicomponent	Presence of globules, reticulation, blotches, dots, veil, regression structures, branched streaks, radial streaming, vascular structures and/or structureless areas (3 or more of these structures need to be present)

Recurrent (persistent) nevi

Definition

Persistent nevi, also called recurrent nevi or "pseudomelanoma", are defined as recurrences of pigmentation that appear after incomplete removal of a compound or intradermal melanocytic nevus. In recurrent nevi, the appearance of the pigmentation usually develops within 6 months from time of initial biopsy. In contrast, recurrence of melanoma characteristically appears years later. In addition, in persistent nevi the pigment almost never extends beyond the scar (i.e. the pigment is usually confined to the center of the scar), whereas in recurrent melanoma the pigment frequently extends beyond the scar. Reactive pigmentation (post inflammatory hyperpigmentation) appears inside the scar and can occur in any surgical scar, independent of the previous existence of a nevus or not. This pigmentation is not caused by persistence of nevus cells.

Dermoscopic criteria

The criteria are asymmetry, sharp borders, homogeneous or multicomponent pattern, atypical pigment network, irregular streaks, black dots, globules, and blue-gray or red colors. The dermoscopic features of persistent nevi are also commonly seen in primary melanoma.

In the case of "reactive pigmentation" of scars, globules are always absent.

5b: Melanoma (Figures A4–A12)

The clinical and dermoscopic appearance of the malignant melanoma depends on the subtype of tumor, its location, the degree of pigmentation, the existence of a previous nevus and the status of progression of the tumor. Most features of melanoma have been reviewed in Chapter 4 (pattern analysis and the different algorithms used to differentiate nevi from melanoma).

The main dermoscopic criteria of malignant melanoma can be summarized into one of three patterns, having some or all of global and local features listed in Box 5.1. In the case of melanomas on special locations (palms, soles, nails and face), different structures have to be recognized (see Chapter 6).

In Figure 5.2 the major findings in benign, suspicious and malignant melanocytic tumors are depicted.

Box 5.1 *Main dermoscopic criteria of melanoma on non-globrous skin*

Global features
■ Asymmetry
■ Multiple colors (tan, dark brown, black, blue-gray, white, red)
Patterns
■ Multicomponent pattern (combination of three or more structures)
■ Starburst pattern in adulthood
■ Non-specific pattern
Local features
■ Atypical pigment network
■ Atypical streaks (pseudopods, radial streaming)
■ Atypical dots/globules
■ Atypical vessels
■ Regression structures
■ Blue-white veil

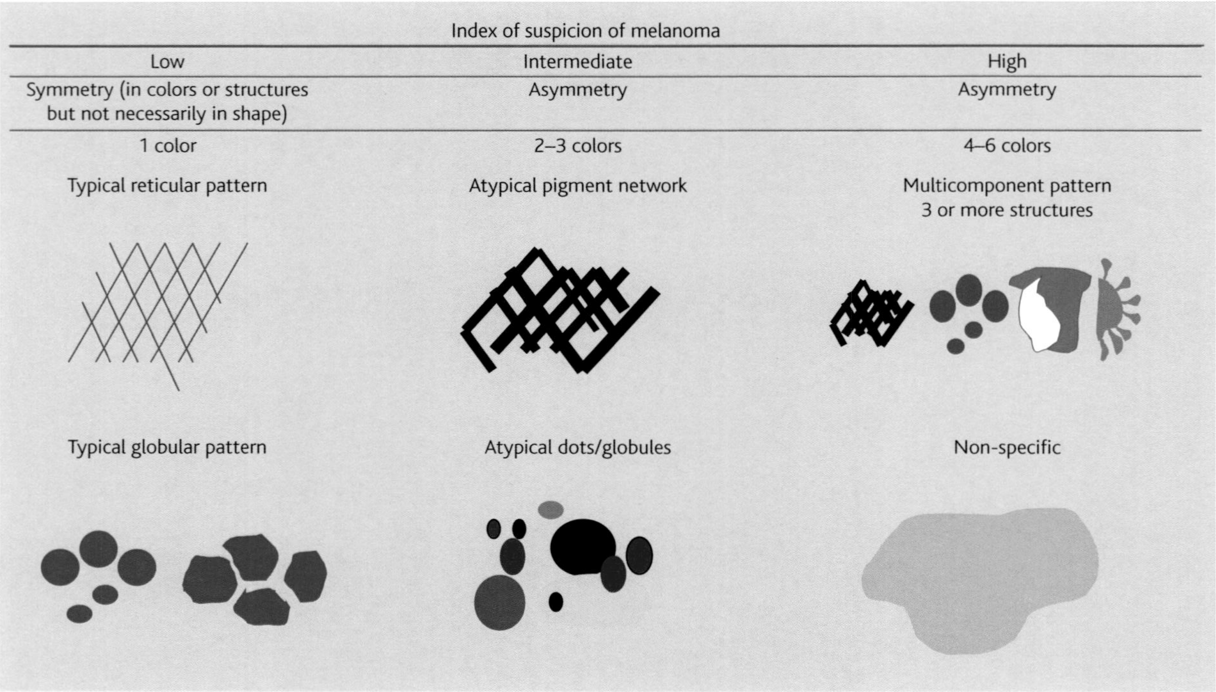

Index of suspicion of melanoma

Low	Intermediate	High
Symmetry (in colors or structures but not necessarily in shape)	Asymmetry	Asymmetry
1 color	2–3 colors	4–6 colors
		Multicomponent pattern 3 or more structures
Typical reticular pattern	Atypical pigment network	
Typical globular pattern	Atypical dots/globules	Non-specific

Figure 5.2 Simplified algorithm of dermoscopic criteria for low, intermediate and high suspicion for melanoma

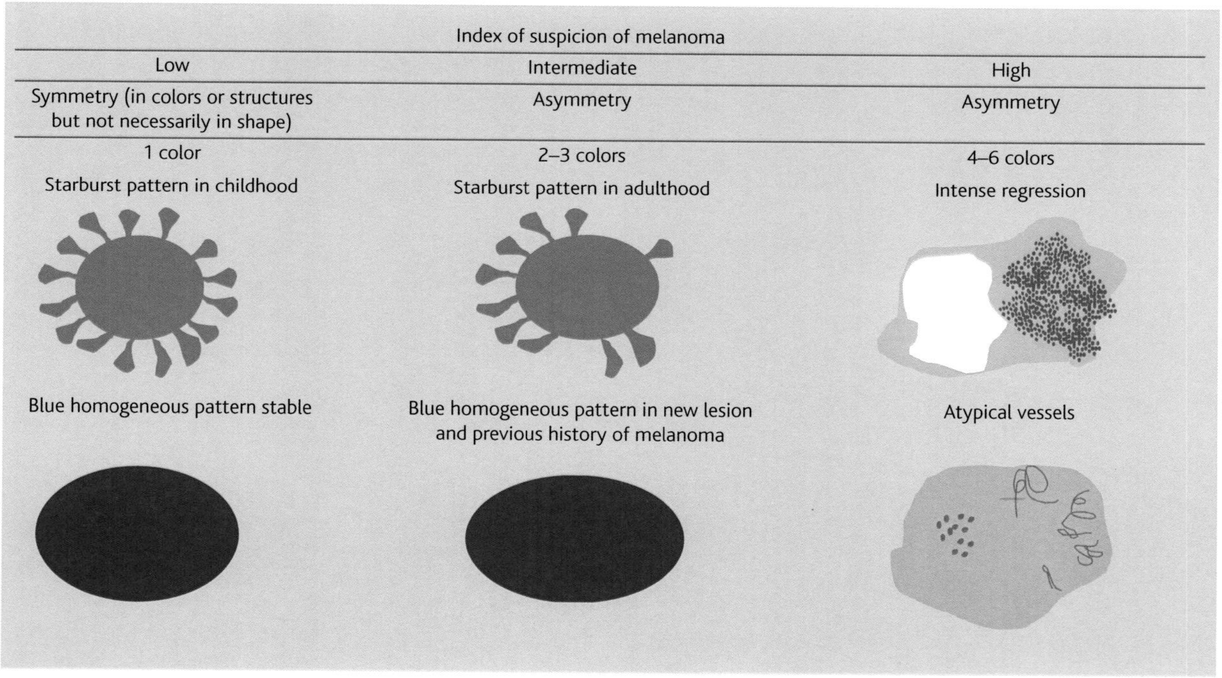

	Index of suspicion of melanoma	
Low	Intermediate	High
Symmetry (in colors or structures but not necessarily in shape)	Asymmetry	Asymmetry
1 color	2–3 colors	4–6 colors
Starburst pattern in childhood	Starburst pattern in adulthood	Intense regression
Blue homogeneous pattern stable	Blue homogeneous pattern in new lesion and previous history of melanoma	Atypical vessels

Figure 5.2 Continued

Special locations

6

6a: Lesions on the face (Figures A11, A12)

Lentigo maligna melanoma (LMM) is increasing in incidence, and the average age at diagnosis decreases year by year. Facial pigmented lesions are a frequent esthetic query in dermatologic practice and some of the lesions can be early LMM. Dermoscopy can be helpful in detecting suspicious patterns and in the selection of the best areas to biopsy to rule out melanoma.

Under dermoscopy, the presence of a pseudonetwork is characteristic of pigmented lesions on the face. This feature is not related to the rete ridges of the epidermis – which are absent or blunted due to the anatomy of the skin in this area and to photoaging – but is due to the interruption of the homogeneous pigmentation by the openings of hair follicle ostia and adnexal structures (Table 6.1)

6b: Lesions on palms and soles (Figures 6.1a–c, A14–18)

Dermoscopy can improve the clinician's diagnostic accuracy when evaluating volar lesions. Acral lentiginous melanoma (ALM) is the most frequent type of melanoma in non-white populations, whearese ALM accounts for about 4.5–7% of all melanomas in white populations. However, the overall incidence in all populations, regardless of race, seems to be equivalent. It is intuitively obvious that the clinical recognition of benign lesions will decrease the number of unnecessary surgeries. In addition, the increase in sensitivity of diagnosing ALM will improve the early detection of this cancer.

Table 6.1 *Lesions on the face*

Dermoscopy patterns	Definition	Schema
Features of lentigo maligna melanoma (LMM)		
Asymmetric pigmented follicular openings	The proliferation of melanocytes in the follicle, characteristic of LMM even in the early stages, result in asymmetric pigmentation of the follicular openings	
Dark rhomboidal structures	Dark pigmentation around follicles forming rhomboidal or polygonal structures. If present, these are highly specific for melanoma	
Slate-gray dots and globules	Multiple slate-gray dots and globules, irregular in size, corresponding to melanophages. Can also be present in lichen planus-like keratosis and actinic keratosis. Some LMM exhibit only this feature	
Homogeneous areas	Complete occlusion of follicular openings due to the melanoma cell invasion of the follicular structures	

Because of the parallel arrangement of ridges and furrows making up the surface skin markings (dermoglyphics), melanocytic lesions on this anatomical site exhibit characteristic parallel patterns different from patterns seen on non-glabrous skin (Figures 6.1a–c, Table 6.2).

Table 6.1 Continued

Dermoscopy patterns	Definition	Schema
Features in benign lesions		
Light brown fingerprint-like areas	Light brown, delicate, network-like structures resembling the pattern of fingerprints. Seen in lentigo	
Keratin pseudocysts	Brown-yellowish, round to oval, sharply circumscribed structures, often displaying a targetoid appearance. Seen in seborrheic keratosis	
Yellow opaque areas	Areas of amorphous yellowish pigmentation corresponding to keratin. Seen in seborrheic keratosis	
Moth-eaten border	Abrupt cut-off with a concave indentation at the border. Seen in lentigo	

6c: Dermoscopic findings of pigmented lesions of the nail apparatus (Figures A19, A20)

Melanonychia striata may be a sign indicating early nail-apparatus melanoma (1% of melanomas). Nail matrix biopsy is usually painful and often leaves permanent nail dystrophy. Dermoscopy provides additional criteria to decide if a nail-apparatus biopsy is necessary (Table 6.3).

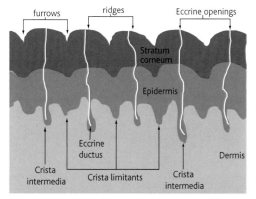

Figure 6.1a Schematic representation of the anatomy of volar skin

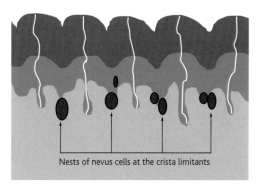

Figure 6.1b Schematic representation of melanocytic nevus

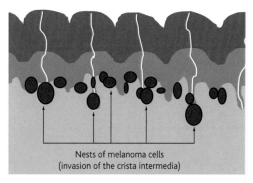

Figure 6.1c Schematic representation of melanoma on volar skin

61

Table 6.2 Lesions on palms and soles

Dermoscopy patterns	Definition	Schema
Benign patterns		
Parallel furrow pattern	Pigmentation following the furrows	
Parallel furrow pattern variants	Parallel furrow pattern with the addition of brown dots or globules following the ridges	
	Brown dots or globules following the ridges	
	Double-lined pigmentation following the furrows	
Lattice-like pattern	Pigmentation following the furrows plus linear bands of pigment crossing from one to the next like rungs of a ladder	
	Only linear bands of pigment crossing the ridges; no furrow pigmentation	

Table 6.2 Continued

Dermoscopy patterns	Definition	Schema
Fibrillar/filamentous pattern[a]	Parallel fine streaks crossing the dermoglyphics in a tangential direction	
Globular pattern	Globules not associated with a parallel pattern	
Homogeneous pattern	Light brown homogeneous pigmentation with an amorphous appearance	
Acral reticular pattern	Well-defined pigment network not associated with the skin markings	
Non-typical pattern	Lesions that cannot be classified into the previous mentioned groups and lack any specific features of malignancy	
Malignant patterns		
Parallel ridge pattern[b]	Linear pigmentation of the ridges	
Diffuse variegate pigmentation	Pigmented blotches of various shades of brown observed in some portions of the lesion	

Table 6.2 Continued

Dermoscopy patterns	Definition	Schema
Serrated pattern	Abrupt edge and streaks at the periphery	
Multicomponent pattern	Abrupt edge, diffuse pigmentation, peripheral irregular globules and dots, multiple colors, atypical streaks in combination with localized areas exhibiting benign patterns (fibrillar, parallel furrow or lattice-like)	
Atypical reticulated/ lattice-like pattern	Present in some superficial-spreading melanomas in volar areas with a broadened pigment network or broadened lattice-like pattern	

[a]Few in-situ melanomas can exhibit a fibrillar pattern with thick lines.
[b]Few active junctional nevi (less than 1%) can exhibit a parallel ridge pattern. The parallel ridge pattern can also be present in racial pigmentation and in macules seen in Peutz–Jeghers syndrome.

Table 6.3 *Lesions of the nail apparatus*

Feature	Schema
Features of melanocytic lesion	
Brown background. The background of the pigmented area is brown with dots and is due to melanin	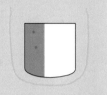
Features indicating nevus	
Brown longitudinal parallel lines that are regular in coloration, spacing and thickness throughout the whole lesion	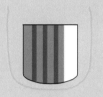
Features indicating melanoma	
Brown to black longitudinal lines, irregular in coloration, spacing and thickness disrupting the normal parallel pattern	
Blood spots in association with criteria of melanocytic lesion. Recent bleeding: purple, round-shaped. Older bleeding: proximal edge sharply demarcated with ovoid or polycyclic border while distal edge appears elongated in a "filamentous pattern"	

Table 6.3 Continued

Feature	Schema
Micro-Hutchinson's sign. Pigmentation of the cuticle invisible to the naked eye	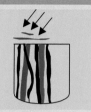
Features indicating non-melanocytic lesions	
Homogeneous grayish lines and gray background: ■ Characteristic of nail apparatus lentigo ■ Drug-induced nail pigmentation ■ Ethnic-type nail pigmentation	

7 Other lesions (Figures A30–A35)

Dermoscopy is a non-invasive procedure mainly developed for evaluating pigmented skin lesions. However, this procedure has been used in other areas of dermatology. Other applications of dermoscopy that are not treated in other chapters of this handbook are summarized in Table 7.1.

Table 7.1 Other applications of dermoscopy

Diseases	Dermoscopic criteria	Schema
Infestations		
Scabies	Gray delta structures and ovoid translucent structures similar to a jet contrail	
Tungiasis	Amorphous yellowish tumors without vessels inside	
Pediculosis	Direct visualization of the parasite and ovoid "nits" on the proximal hair	

Table 7.1 Continued

Diseases	Dermoscopic criteria	Schema
Infections		
Molluscum contagiosum	Polylobular whitish-yellowish amorphous structure in the center of the lesions with surrounding crown of vessels, some of them branching, which do not cross the center of the lobules (also called "red corona")	
Verrucae	Red globules with whitish halo corresponding to thrombosed capillaries	
Other malignant tumors		
Bowen's disease (squamous cell carcinoma)	Clusters of glomerular vessels and scaly surface	
Other tumors		
Keratoacanthoma	Hairpin vessels with whitish halo and central hyperkeratosis	

Table 7.1 Continued

Diseases	Dermoscopic criteria	Schema
Clear cell acanthoma	Red globules arranged in a pattern that resembles a string of pearls	
Lichen planus-like keratosis	Brownish gray and bluish gray, localized or diffuse, coarse granules in the absence of specific criteria of melanocytic lesion	
Sebaceous gland hyperplasia	Aggregated white or yellow papules surrounded by groups of orderly winding, scarcely branching vessels that may extend towards the center but which do not cross over the center	
Collision or compound tumors	Presence of two or more different lesions, each showing its own specific dermoscopic features	
Inflammatory diseases Psoriasis	Homogeneous red dots with some patches of pink to bright red (dotted vessels)	

Table 7.1 Continued

Diseases	Dermoscopic criteria	Schema
Lichen planus	■ Diffuse structureless, brownish areas ■ Fine or coarse gray-blue or brown dots or globules ■ Wickhams striae and vessels	
Lichen aureus	Red-coppery color of the background, with round to oval red dots, globules and patches, gray dots and a partial grayish network	
Porokeratosis	A "white tract" structure surrounding nearly the entire perimeter of the lesion, and brownish pigmentation in the central portion. Some areas reveal the classic "double tract" of scale with double white line that corresponds to "cornoid lamella"	
Vascular lesions (excluding angiomas)		
Subcorneal or intracutaneous hematoma in acral skin	Dark red to black homogeneous areas with some black-reddish globules at the periphery. In black heel, black-reddish globules on the ridges (resembling pebbles) are characteristic	

Table 7.1 *Continued*

Diseases	Dermoscopic criteria	Schema
Subungual Hematoma	Purple coloration of the pigmentation with an elongated parallel linear pattern at the distal edge and a well-demarcated round-shaped proximal edge. A characteristic features is the presence of blood spots at the proximal end of the nail (pebbles)	
Stasis dermatitis	Glomerular vessels and scaly surface	

Further reading

Argenziano G, Soyer HP, De Giorgi V, et al. Interactive atlas of dermoscopy. Milan: Edra Medical Publishing and New Media, 2000. (book and CD-ROM).

Blum A, Kreusch JF, Bauer J, Garbe C (eds). Dermatoskopie von Hauttumoren mit interaktiver. Darmstadt: Steinkopff Verlag, 2003. (CD-ROM).

Cabo H. Dermatoscopia. Buenos Aires: Weber Ferro, Medios Interactivos, 2000. (CD-ROM).

Johr R, Soyer HP, Argenziano G, Hofmann-Wellenhof R, Scalvenzi M. Dermoscopy: the essentials. Edinburgh: Mosby, 2004.

Kreusch J, Rassner G. Auflichtmikroskopie pigmentierter Hauttumoren. Ein Bildatlas. Stuttgart: Thieme, 1991.

Malvehy J, Puig S (eds). Principles of dermoscopy. Barcelona: CEGE Editors, 2002.

Marghoob AA, Braun PR, Kopf AW (eds). Atlas of dermoscopy. London: Taylor & Francis, 2005.

Menzies SW, Crotty KA, Ingvar C, McCarthy WH. An atlas of surface microscopy of pigmented skin lesions: dermoscopy, 2nd edn. Roseville: McGraw-Hill Australia, 2003.

Rabinovitz HS. Dermoscopy. A practical guide. Miami: MMA Worldwide Group Inc, 1999. (CD-ROM).

Rabinovitz HS, Cognetta JR. AB. Dermoscopy and new imaging techniques. Dermatology Clinics, Philadelphia: WB Saunders, 2001.

Soyer HP, Argenziano G, Chimenti S, et al. Dermoscopy of pigmented skin lesions. An atlas based on the Consensus Net Meeting on Dermoscopy 2000. Milan: Edra Medical Publishing and New Media, 2001.

Stolz W, Braun-Falco O, Bilek P, et al. Color atlas of dermatoscopy, 2nd edn. Berlin: Blackwell Publishing, 2002.

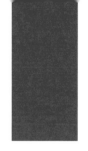

Appendix

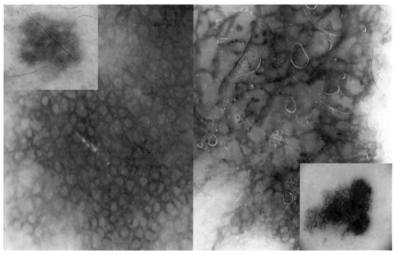

Figure A1 *Pigment network in melanocytic tumors (CPL). Typical pigment network in a junctional nevus (left) and atypical pigment network in a in situ malignant melanoma (right).*

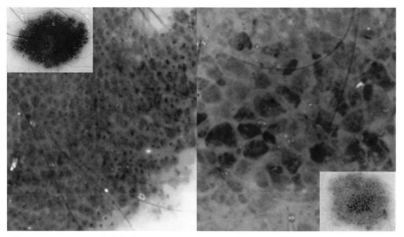

Figure A2 *Variants of globular pattern in compound nevi. Cobblestone pattern is seen on the right.*

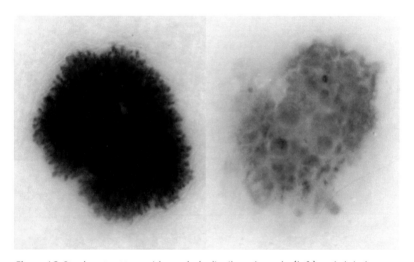

Figure A3 *Star burst pattern with regularly distributed streaks (left) and globular pattern (right) in Spitz/Reed nevi (CPL).*

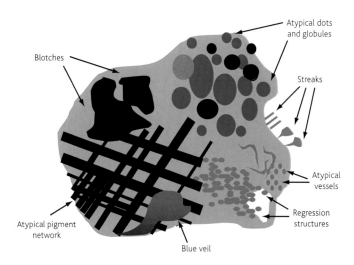

Figure A4 Dermoscopic structures in malignant melanoma.

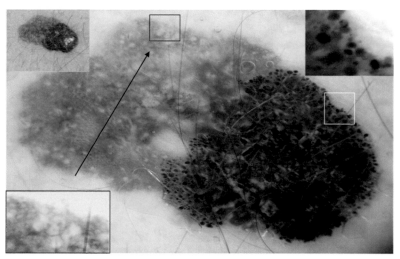

Figure A5 Superficial spreading malignant melanoma (CPL). Multicomponent pattern, multiple colors (black, dark and light brown, blue-gray, red, white). Atypical network (black box) and globules/dots (white box), blue dots and white structureless areas due to regression. TDS (Total Dermoscop Score) = $2 \times 1.3 + 4 \times 0.1 + 6 \times 0.5 + 5 \times 0.5 = 8.5$

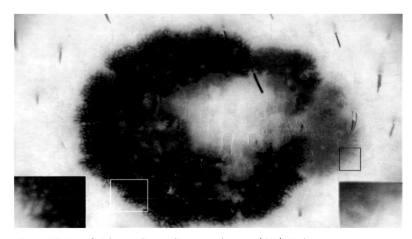

Figure A6 *Superficial spreading malignant melanoma (CPL). Multicomponent pattern, asymmetry in two axes and multiple colors (black, dark and light brown, blue-gray, white). Atypical network and streaks are visible at the periphery (squares show magnification). Irregular black blotches in combination with blue dots and white structureless areas due to regression in the center of the tumor. TDS= 2 × 1.3 + 6 × 0.1 + 5 × 0.5 + 3 × 0.5 = 7.2*

Figure A7 *Superficial spreading malignant melanoma (CPL). Multicomponent pattern, asymmetry in two axes and multiple colors (black, dark and light brown, blue-gray). Irregular streaks are visible at the periphery. Irregular dots/globules and blotches in combination with blue dots due to regressions are visible in the center of the tumor. TDS= 2 × 1.3 + 4 × 0.1 + 4 × 0.5 + 3 × 0.5 = 6.5*

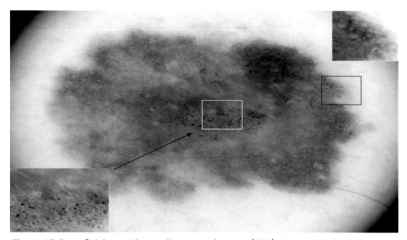

Figure A8 Superficial spreading malignant melanoma (CPL). Asymmetry in two axes, multiple colors (black, dark and light brown, blue-gray) and multicomponent pattern composed of globules (white box), pigment network and homogeneous areas. Atypical globules and regression structures (blue dots) are seen in the center. Atypical pigment network is present at the periphery of the tumor (black box). TDS= $1.3 \times 2 + 1 \times 0.1 + 4 \times 0.5 + 4 \times 0.5 = 6.7$

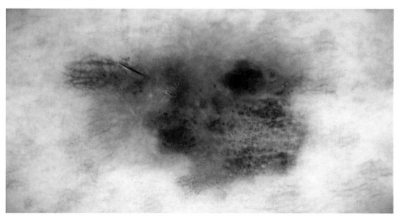

Figure A9 Superficial spreading malignant melanoma (CPL). Multicomponent pattern (globules, pigment network and homogeneous areas) with asymmetry in two axes and multiple colors (black, dark and light brown, red and blue-gray). Atypical globules and dots (brown and black), atypical network, branched streaks and regression structures (scar-like areas and blue-gray dots) are present in the tumor. TDS= $1.3 \times 2 + 0.1 \times 3 + 5 \times 0.5 + 5 \times 0.5 = 7.9$

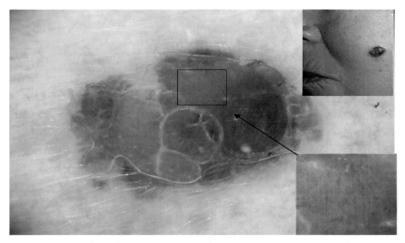

Figure A10 Nodular melanoma with atypical large nests containing atypical vessels (magnification) and blue-white veil and milky-red area (CPL).

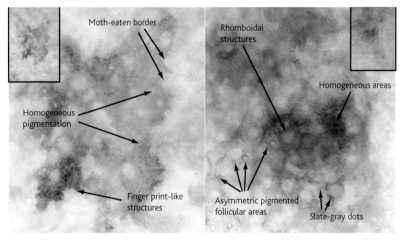

Figure A11 Lentigo solaris (left) on the face with Moth eaten border, homogeneous pigmentation and finger print structures (CPL). Lentigo maligna melanoma (right) exhibiting asymmetric pigmented follicular areas, slate-gray dots, homogeneous areas and rhomboidal structures (CPL).

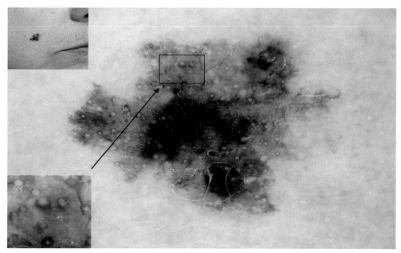

Figure A12 *In situ malignant melanoma (lentigo maligna melanoma) (CPL). Asymmetric pigmentation of the folicular openings, rhomboidal structures and occlusion of the follicular openings.*

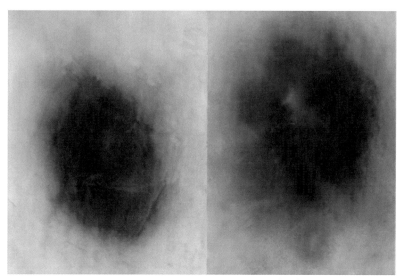

Figure A13 *Homogeneous blue pigmentation in blue nevus (left) and metastasis of melanoma (right) (CPL).*

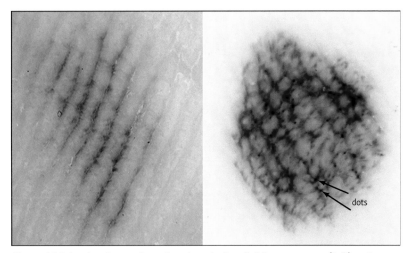

Figure A14 *Acral melanocytic nevi on the sole. Parallel furrow pattern (left) and lattice-like pattern (right).*

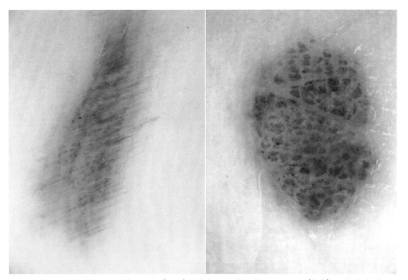

Figure A15 *Acral nevi on the sole (CPL) exhibiting fibrillar pattern (left) and globular pattern (right).*

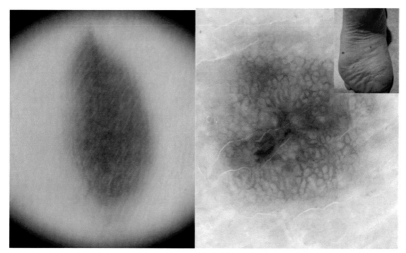

Figure A16 *Acral congenital nevus (CPL) exhibiting blue homogeneous pattern (left) and acquired nevus on the sole with a reticular pattern (right).*

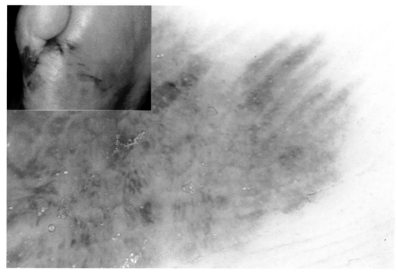

Figure A17 *Acral lentiginous melanoma. Parallel ridge pattern and difuse pigmentation.*

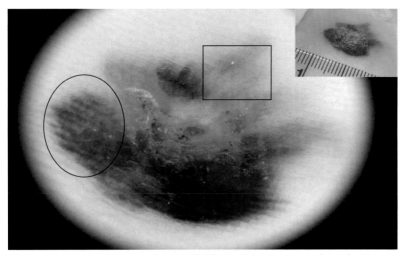

Figure A18 *Acral lentiginous melanoma (CPL). Parallel ridge pattern (circle), difuse irregular pigmentation (square) and ulceration in the center.*

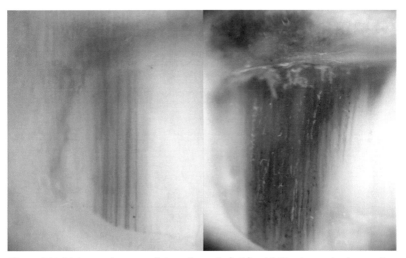

Figure A19 *Melanocytic nevus of the nail matrix (left) exhibiting brown background and brown longitudinal parallel lines regular in coloration, spacing and thickness through the whole lesion (CPL). Melanoma of the nail matrix (right) with Hutchingson's sign, brown background and brown longitudinal parallel lines irregular in coloration, spacing and thickness through the whole lesion (CPL).*

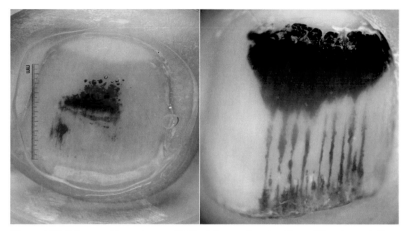

Figure A20 Subungual hematoma with black to purple coloration of the pigmentation with an elongated parallel linear pattern at the distal edge and a well demarcated round-shaped proximal edge with a characteristic feature of blood spots (pebbles).

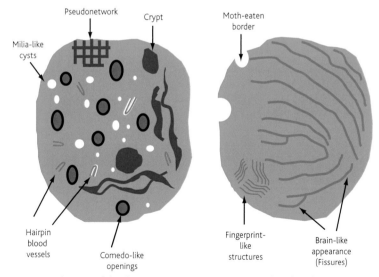

Figure A21 Schaema of the dermoscopic structures seen in seborrheic keratosis.

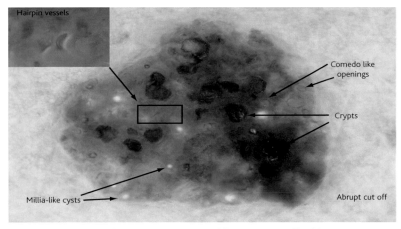

Figure A22 Sebhorreic keratosis with comedo-like openings, millia-like cysts, crypts, fissures and hairpin vessels (magnification) with white halo (CPL).

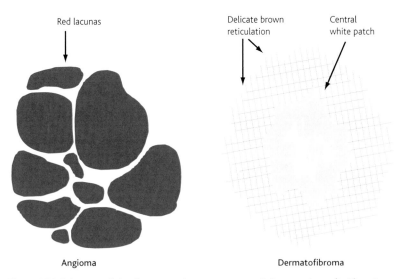

Figure A23 Schaema of the dermoscopic structures seen in hemangioma (left) and dermatofibroma (right).

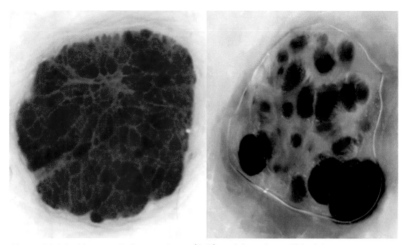

Figure A24 Red lagoons in hemangioma (left) and thrombosed black lagoons in angiokeratoma (right).

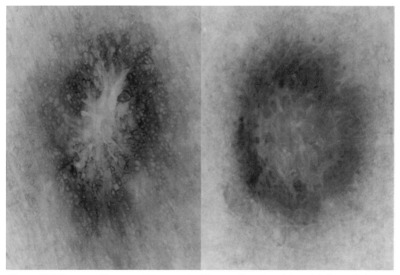

Figure A25 Dermatofibroma with central white patch and peripheral delicate light brown reticulation (left). When viewed under polarized dermoscopy, the central scar-like area appears pink (right) (CPL).

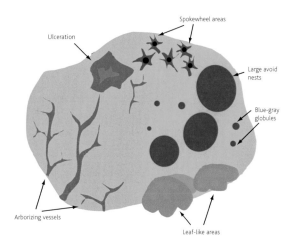

Figure A26 *Schaema of the dermoscopic structures seen in basal cell carcinoma.*

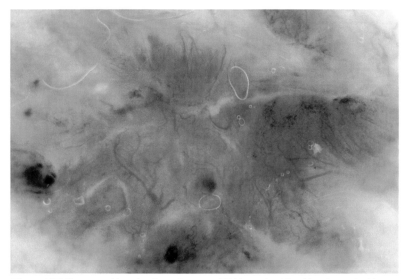

Figure A27 *Pigmented basal cell carcinoma exhibiting arborizing blood vessels, blue-gray globules and large blue-gray nests (CPL).*

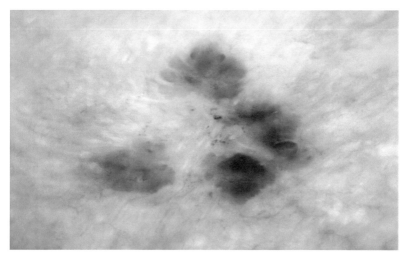

Figure A28 *Basal cell carcinoma exhibiting leaf-like structures, arborizing blood vessels, large blue ovoid nests and blue-gray globules (CPL). In the centre, one can also see a "shiny white structureless area".*

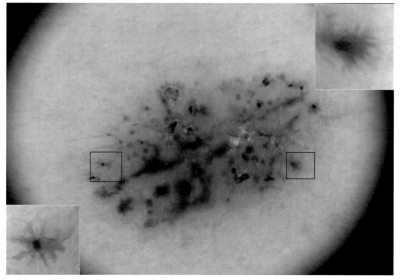

Figure A29 *Basal cell carcinoma exhibiting spoke-wheel structures (magnification), ulceration, large ovoid nests and blue-gray globules (CPL).*

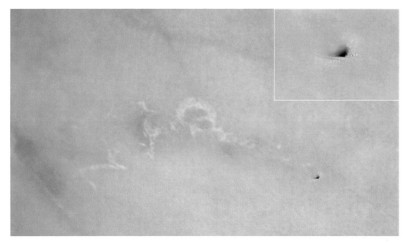

Figure A30 *Scabies with gray delta structures at the begining of the "sulcus" corresponding to the parasite and ovoid translucent structures similar to a jet contrail (CPL).*

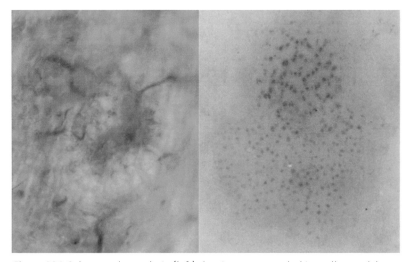

Figure A31 *Sebaceous hyperplasia (left) showing aggregated white-yellow nodules surrounded by groups of orderly winding, scarcely branching blood vessels that extend towards the center without crossing it (CPL). The lesion on the right has red globules forming a string of pearls, a characteristic of clear cell acanthoma (CPL).*

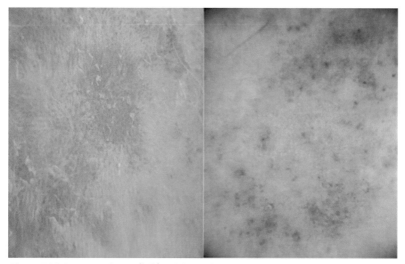

Figure A32 *Psoriasis plaque (left) exhibiting homogeneous red globule vessels with hyperkeratosis (CPL). Diffuse glomerular vessels in stasis dermatitis (right) (CPL).*

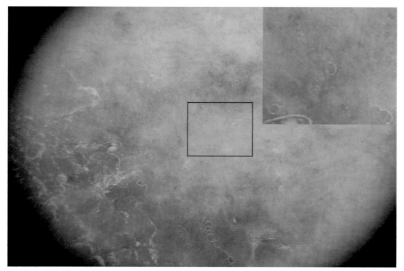

Figure A33 *Bowen disease (squamous cell carcinoma in situ) with clusters of glomerular vessels (square) and keratin in the absense of specific criteria for melanocytic lesion (CPL).*

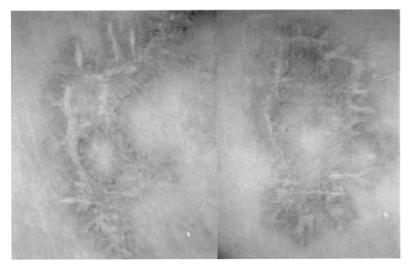

Figure A34 *Lichen planus with Wickham striae and vessels seen under dermoscopic examination (CPL).*

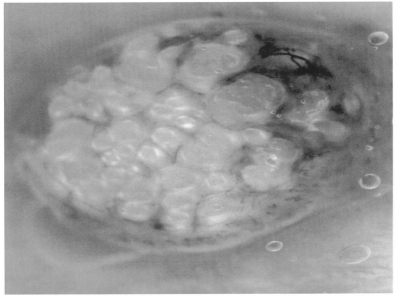

Figure A35 *Dermoscopy of moluscum contagiosum (CPL).*

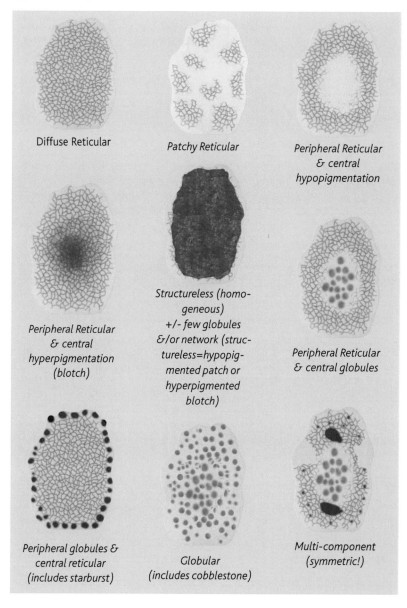

Diffuse Reticular

Patchy Reticular

Peripheral Reticular & central hypopigmentation

Peripheral Reticular & central hyperpigmentation (blotch)

Structureless (homogeneous) +/- few globules &/or network (structureless=hypopigmented patch or hyperpigmented blotch)

Peripheral Reticular & central globules

Peripheral globules & central reticular (includes starburst)

Globular (includes cobblestone)

Multi-component (symmetric!)

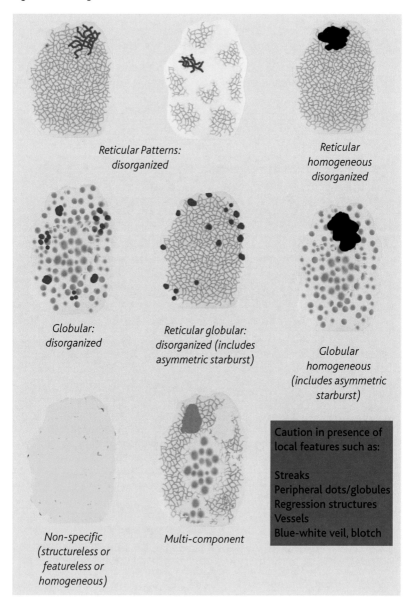

Reticular Patterns:
disorganized

Reticular
homogeneous
disorganized

Globular:
disorganized

Reticular globular:
disorganized (includes
asymmetric starburst)

Globular
homogeneous
(includes asymmetric
starburst)

Non-specific
(structureless or
featureless or
homogeneous)

Multi-component

Caution in presence of
local features such as:

Streaks
Peripheral dots/globules
Regression structures
Vessels
Blue-white veil, blotch

Index

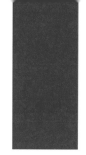

Page numbers in italics represent tables, figures and boxes.

Printed and bound by CPI Group (UK) Ltd, Croydon, CR0 4YY

01/11/2024

01782637-0001